Surviving Cancer:

A Holistic Approach To Healing

Copyright © 2016

By John Baez

Printed in USA

ISBN-13: 978-1523620340
ISBN-10: 152362034X

Acknowledgements

I am thankful for the journey that made these words possible,

The technology that has allowed it to reach you,

The numerous authors that all contributed to my understanding,

The many people that believed in me and made this a part of their journey,

And to the special people in my life:

Melinda, for listening and always inspiring me,

My daughter Michel, for teaching me to be a better father,

And my grand daughter Milani, for keeping the child in me alive.

Contents

I was inspired to write this because:

"Writers change the world one reader at a time. But you can't change the world with a book that's still on your hard drive or in a box under your bed."

Joel Friedlander – The Book Designer

"The 'i' in illness is isolation, and the crucial letters in wellness is 'we'."

Author unknown

Forward

It was during a dive trip that I felt my first pangs of pain. I thought it might be my activities so I slowed down a bit and gave it no further thought. But it kept coming back. A few days later the pain had grown significantly. It would hit me in bouts for about a minute every 20-30 minutes, all day.

That was my body's alarm; telling me something was very wrong. I visited the doctor and an hour later I was given the news, I had testicular cancer.

Looking back I realize how life had prepared me for this moment. I had a friend that was an oncology nurse, meditated, was health conscious (or so I thought), and aware that 'I was what I ate' (and was I).

I had never really been sick before. Through my ordeal I learned a lot about orthodox medicine and found that today's medical practices are a sad state of affairs. I consulted various specialists, and not one of them really cared to help me. They all just went about suggesting the same thing and predicting the same, grim, outcome. Not one of them took any interest in why I might have become sick. Not one of them hinted that something in my life might have caused this. 'It just happens' was the attitude.

I am fortunate. I love to read and had read many stories. For some unknown reason I had always been curious about sickness and healing. My oncology friend and what she'd seen throughout her years at work made it clear to me that chemotherapy and radiation would just finish killing me. My philosophy on life told me that I had caused this. It wasn't just something that 'happens'. My understanding of the body told me that I could get myself out of this.

You are holding in your hands the result of my journey, everything I learned, the things that heal, the amazing capability of the human body, how it changed me, the amazing people that taught me, all that gives me life today. I learned to live as we are intended to live on this planet.

I have hope for change. We don't have to be sick, none of us. Today I don't even get colds. It begins with awareness, understanding our nature and place on this planet, having respect for our environment and the evolutionary process that has been in place for eons.

I give thanks for what I've learned, for everyone that has been a part of this journey and for the ability to, and privilege of, sharing it with you today. You WILL heal. Here is a way to guide you...

Introduction

Being diagnosed with a life threatening disease is one of the scariest things that can occur to anyone. When it happened to me I felt alone and confused. No advisor I found was helpful. The variety of opinions immediately convinced me that amidst all of this confusion I could not really count on anyone. It was 1996. At the age of 37 my life flashed before me. I had cancer (testicular cancer, spread to lymph nodes, lungs and brain; I was told at this stage I could live about a year because 'I was strong').

I will always recall the day like yesterday. I knew things weren't good when I walked into the doctor's office. I had been in pain for days. I was almost overcome by fear and anger when I heard the diagnosis (which I already knew was the case based on my symptoms). As he was laying out my course of therapy (without even consulting me he assumed I'd be hospitalized for surgery immediately followed by 'chemo') I told him he had no right to take away my hope and that even though I was not well I expected that I would be. I got up and left in a 'fearful rage'.

It is now 2015 as I write this so obviously I survived. I am stronger and healthier now (at 55) than I have ever been at a time when many people are considered passed their prime. I intend to stay that way for many years to come and have learned that this is how it should be if we live as we should. This is my story, what I've learned and how my journey has stretched out to help others whose lives have crossed mine.

Who I am (no one special) is not as important as what I am giving you. What you do with this information is completely up to you. Just so you know, I am 100% percent certain that, regardless of your circumstances, this will help you. I have helped and watched many people return to life over the years. That is why (and at the request of a few friends) I am writing this.

As you read keep in mind that your wellbeing is 100% up to you and only you. No doctor can heal you; no medication is a silver bullet and no one knows you and your circumstances like you do. At most others can guide you and support your journey... but only you can heal yourself. And, regardless of what any expert says, YOU CAN.

The basis for health lies in understanding. Modern day life conflicts with our biological nature and what our body requires to be healthy. We are not meant to be unhealthy. It is the impact of modern living that brings disease into our lives. Humanity is out of control and in a state of confusion. We are our own worse enemy. The secret to life and health is in harmonizing with the ways of nature.

Observe and you will see that humans are the only living beings on this planet that live against their nature. We act and eat in ways that are completely unnatural and against our biological nature. We have this belief that we are more capable than our environment and the evolutionary process so we are constantly modifying it (with severe consequences). Ever since the advent of agriculture we have been attempting to alter our environment and ourselves.

This, as we'll see, is the basis for a great many of our problems.

In all fairness, not everything we do is detrimental! Indeed some of our modern day advances are amazing. But when it comes to anything affecting our biology and health such as food preparation, hygiene, medicine, our environment and life's motive itself we would do ourselves a great service if we stopped, revisited the status-quo and what we're doing, and went back to basics.

It is beyond the scope of this book to get into these topics in detail. More than likely they would each require a book in and of themselves. But it is important to understand that if you are sick you are likely a victim of modern humanity. You may be wondering why this has happened to you, what you have done, why modern medicine is not helping you. Hopefully you will develop an understanding. And that understanding will help you on your journey.

Many books have been written that discuss what I am discussing here. However, there is a lot of information that needs to be sorted out. My hope is that I can contribute to sorting out a few things such that you have a guide that helps you to heal and possibly enhance other

> "Health is worth more than learning."
> Thomas Jefferson

aspects of being human. There is plenty of (well intended) stuff out there but where do you start? How do you know what's right for you? Just go

4

to your local bookstore (or online) and look at the number of volumes in the 'self help', 'nutrition' and 'medical' sections. If you are sick you don't necessarily have time for all this research. That is a major reason for this volume. When I discovered books as a young man I sought them out to guide me in finding answers to every question I had. I was somewhat disappointed when I learned that there was no guidebook for being human. When I became ill I realized that my body was telling me that something needed to change. It turns out that it has been a very worthwhile journey. Today I am sharing the results with you.

We are always hearing the word 'health' tossed around. Yet most of us only have an implied and distorted meaning of what it really means to be healthy. Here in the US, the media is busy trying to give you an understanding that is largely to their (financial) benefit (it's that greed/selfish

> "Healing may not be so much about getting better, as about letting go of everything that isn't you – all of the expectations, all of the beliefs – and becoming who you are."
> Rachel Naomi Remen

thing rearing it's ugly head) rather than really helping you to understand what it is to be healthy and how to get there. The medical industry itself is regulated by money (insurance and pharmaceuticals actually control much of how treatments are administered and only favor treatments that are financially lucrative) with the patient placed a far second after stockholders. If your definition of health is based on the system/media then you are likely in for a big surprise. Here we will clarify once and for all what health is and how you play the primary role in achieving and maintaining it.

The great majority of people I've helped had some form of cancer. However, this is an approach to being healthy and will aid you in healing from many ailments. What we are doing here is giving the body an optimal environment for creating health. This will help you under any circumstance.

My experience, lessons, and recommendations are broken down into various areas in an effort to keep some sense of organization. The book is deliberately short and, hopefully, simple to read. I apologize in advance for any confusion my rambling may bring. Others have successfully used excerpts of this writing so I hope you will understand and use it as well.

Immediate Actions

"Realize that now, in this precise moment of time, you are creating.
You are creating your next moment."

Sara Paddison

If you are ill with a life-threatening ailment (cancer, for example) you have to take action immediately. While it is important to understand the 'why' of everything I recommend it is more important that you take action immediately as time is critical. The following paragraphs outline what to do in order to start healing. In later sections I'll explain why these things are important and will give you additional references and comments. But first the basics; there are 3 areas of change that you MUST undertake immediately.

The first area is dietary. You may have heard that 'you are what you eat'. This is very true. You have probably been poisoning and under nourishing yourself for many years without knowing it. Modern food is mostly garbage, filled with additives and processed beyond the body's ability to recognize and process it. Even if you think you are eating well by purchasing your groceries at a 'health food store' you are not doing as well as you think (you are sick after all). I will outline precisely what to eat throughout the day along with guidelines for making food choices.

Second is lifestyle. This is an area of general guidelines around habits that you may have to change. You may need some mental adjustments (seriously) or perhaps to work less or even to change jobs (you'll see why). There are a variety of lifestyle patterns that have been associated with disease. Your body is telling you that something is wrong and that means that changes are required.

Finally you'll have to make changes that I call environmental. These include changes around the house (household products used for cleaning, soap, etc.) and around you (if you live with or are around smokers, for example, exposed to toxic fumes).

If you find any of these things drastic or beyond you then I wish you the best as you go through your journey. In my experience changes in all of the above areas are required to regain health, especially from the life threatening diseases like cancer.

6

Why such change? Essentially, disease, in any form, is your body sounding an alarm that it is not coping well with something in **YOUR** life/environment. All disease is a form of cellular malfunction[1]. And cellular malfunction (excluding trauma) is caused by environmental factors that are from one or more (usually all) of the three areas mentioned. Any remedy that doesn't address the real reason why you are sick is not addressing the problem, only the symptoms. That is why most medical solutions don't work (they may for a short time, but without changing any of the above the disease usually reappears).

Given the proper conditions the body is amazingly capable of recovering from many diseases. That is what we are doing here, creating the most favorable conditions for your body to recover.

There is no silver bullet. As much as we like the idea of ingesting some magic potion to heal us of our ailments it just doesn't work that way. That is why our medical system is failing. There are exceptions for some ailments but none of these are in the chronic category. Our medical system is also quite good at dealing with trauma. But it fails miserably when it comes to systemic disease. The only way to heal a mistreated body is to treat it well. Someday this will be clear to all of us and will become the standard way of treating illness.

Having said this I cannot tell you to start or stop any medical treatment. I will only say that in my experiences, people heal in spite of treatment and not because of it. Chemotherapy and radiation in particular are poisons, aiming to heal the body by destroying it. In most cases they fail. But they are a profitable business that keeps those involved blind. This is where I tell you to consult your doctor before making any changes. If you do consult a doctor, try to find a good one. Hint: If they refuse to listen and help you by working with you, they are not a good one.

Being ill with a life threatening disease is a trying experience that you cannot avoid. Your body is miraculous and, given the right circumstances, will heal itself. These guidelines have worked many times so I deliver them to you confidently.

Diet
Possibly the largest impact on (chronic) disease is your diet. Your body is constantly recycling itself. Cells live for short periods and are

---

[1] For a great layman's explanation of cellular malfunction refer to 'Never Be Sick Again' by Raymond Francis.

constantly renewed. If the nutrients required to maintain and renew cells are not present cells will function poorly and in undesirable ways.

The following recommendations have been fine tuned and refined over many years to provide the body with everything needed to renew itself optimally. Overall, eating is similar for any disease, as the body just needs optimal nourishment to heal itself. Where there are specific recommendations for specific issues it is noted.

The recipes are all at the end of the book in Appendix A.

Meal	Food	Preparation/Notes
Upon rising	Anti-parasite remedy or ACV/lemon water	When on the tincture program use it, otherwise drink ACV/Lemon water
Breakfast	4 oz. fat free cottage cheese w/1 tbsp. flax seed oil (with lignans) and borage oil	Mix together. May add cinnamon and can be mixed with old-fashioned oatmeal if desired.
or	Seedmeal recipe	Once or twice a week.
	Green juice recipe	Follow instructions on how to prepare green juice.
Mid morning	Homemade vegetable broth with seaweed	
Lunch	Organic salad w/cooked sprouted beans	
or	Steamed vegetables w/tofu	Once or twice a week. Use only organic tofu.
Mid afternoon	Black bean soup w/seaweed	
or	Home made vegetable broth w/seaweed	
Dinner	Lentil soup w/sardines[2]	Prepare raw lentils as per instructions and have as much as you like. Note: consume the sardines **only** every 2 days!!!!
or	Cooked beans (your choice) w/mixed vegetables	ON non-sardine days.
Bedtime	ACV/lemon water	
Throughout the day	Green tea	Enjoy this or other teas as outlines in appendix A throughout the day.

You may note that the diet is rather simple and repeats the same foods often. This is deliberate and intended to make it easy to establish a

---

[2] Sardines are the only animal food that is acceptable during healing. If you don't like sardines you can remove it but you are removing a very amazing food.

routine. Over time, as you heal, other choices will become available to you. But for the next few months this will be your food regime.

Water

Water is the most important ingredient you will consume. You will only consume filtered water in glass, ceramic or stainless containers. You will drink at least 10 glasses of water each day (and night). Take notice, absolutely NO plastics. As a matter of fact if you have any plastic containers used for food you will do yourself a favor by getting rid of them all. There is NO safe plastic for food consumption[3].

Cleanse

In addition to the above you will do what today is called the anti-parasite cleanse[4]. Today this cleanse is commercially available. When I was sick it wasn't and I had to make it from scratch. In its commercial form it is called a 'parasite' cleanse but that doesn't matter. What matters is that it is critical to treatment and a must. I still do this cleanse regularly (in its maintenance form) to this date.

The parasite cleanse can be purchased at **www.drclarkstore.com**. It is referred to as the 'parasite-cleanse' and consists of black walnut hull tincture, wormwood capsules and cloves. The tincture comes in powdered/capsule form but I suggest using the liquid form. I've never had anyone use the powdered form so I don't know if it is as effective as the original liquid tincture. I suggest you take it as outlined in Appendix A. (over the years the form of consumption has changed. I can only attest to the manner in which it has worked in my experience).

Green Tea

Feel free to consume organic green tea as desired. It is important to purchase organic green tea and to prepare it correctly as outlined in appendix A. You may sweeten it with pure stevia or agave. You may also add other herbs for flavor as outlined in appendix A.

Nutritional Supplements

In an ideal world the use of supplements would not be required. When our soil was rich and abundant in nutrients it was likely possible to obtain much of our nutrition from the food we ate. I can't confirm this, as I've never lived when that was a true statement. What I know is that today we have plenty of evidence of the power of some nutrients when used as

---

[3] Studies have been conducted testing plastics for toxins. No plastic has been found to be safe.
[4] The anti-parasite cleanse from Dr. Hulda Clarke is a critical part of healing and must be undertaken as indicated immediately.

supplements to our food intake. The following recommendations are the result of extensive self-experimenting, research and observed experiential effects on others.

Supplement	Dose
Coenzyme B-Complex	1 w/breakfast 1 at bedtime
CoQ10 – 100mg	1 w/breakfast
ALA-ALC	1 w/breakfast 1 at bedtime
Selenomethionine – 200mcg.	1 at bedtime
Zinc picolinate – 50mg.	1 at bedtime
Chromium polynicotinate 200mcg.	1 w/breakfast 1 at bedtime
Ester-C – 500mg.	1 w/breakfast 1 at bedtime
Omega 3-6-9 – 1200mg.	2 w/breakfast 2 at bedtime
MSM Sulfur/Flax oil	1 w/breakfast 1 at bedtime

If you are over 40 years old:

Supplement	Dose
DHEA – 25mg.	1 w/breakfast 1 at bedtime
Melatonin – 10mg.	1 at bedtime

Lifestyle

Along with dietary changes it is likely that you will have to change your lifestyle. Changes can range from simple and relatively straightforward to major changes requiring a big commitment. Again, you are sick for a reason and in every case I've ever worked with lifestyle has had something to do with it.

Further in the book I provide a variety of methods that may be helpful to you. If you are serious about healing you must commit yourself and these suggestions will more than likely help you.

Definite Musts

To heal you must form healing habits. These are the habits that lead to a healthy lifestyle. Of all the habits that you might make for yourself there are some that are required when you are sick.

The Don'ts

There are some changes that are non-negotiable. In plain English, stop or die.

No smoking

Smoking tops the list. Just one cigarette negates every possible health benefit you can derive from everything here. It's that simple. You must stop smoking immediately. No patches, no cutting down. You must stop. Chapter 4 provides a few pointers and ways of dealing with the cravings.

No Drugs

Aside from any prescribed medications (and even these are dubious) you must not do any type of drugs. Any drug alters the body's state of balance. Aside from this the delivery mechanism of drugs carry toxins, all of which stress the body and inhibit the healing process. This is true for over the counter drugs as well.

As per prescription drugs the goal is to get off of them if possible[5]. You should talk with your doctor. If it is a good doctor he will understand and work with you to achieve your goals. Otherwise I suggest you get another doctor. If you are addicted to any form of drug please refer to appendix D for an approach to detoxing.

No Junk Food

Any form of food or drink that is not on the Dietary requirements must be avoided. No exceptions. Modern food is the number one source of toxins in the body and leads to the majority of chronic disease. If it is packaged in any way you should not consume it. There are some exceptions and these are noted in the texts.

The Do's

You will likely require changes to make a healthy lifestyle conducive to healing. Your lifestyle contributes to your health and predisposes you to illness or health.

Relax

Stress weakens the body and makes you vulnerable. If you are sick you are likely going through bouts of uncertainty and anxiety. If on top of that you are the provider for your household or are yourself a caregiver you have additional stress. Add to that a stressful job and other life situations and it is easy to see why the body breaks down. This is not a natural

---

[5] I have worked with cases where prescription medications are required for life. Please be informed about any medications you take and why you take it.

11

state that we are designed to cope with. Therefore it is imperative that you learn to relax consciously.

Take time throughout the day, 4 or 5 times each day for 10-15 minutes each time, to consciously relax. Find a quiet place where you will not be interrupted, sit (or lay) comfortably and just focus on breathing. Visualize yourself healing and freeing yourself of disease and stress with every exhalation. Be aware of what ails you and let it go. We go into this in detail in chapter 4. For now use these simple guidelines to get started.

Castor Oil Packs
Each evening, either before showering or before bed, you will administer a castor oil heat pack to yourself. This pack is magical and is based on the healing remedies of Edgar Cayce[6]. Prepare the pack as outlined in Appendix A.

The pack can be applied while lying on your back. Apply for at least 30 minutes daily. Raise the heating pad heat gradually over a period of 5-10 minutes until it is high with care not to burn yourself! The heat helps the skin absorb the castor oil and is very soothing. It should not be uncomfortable.

If you have any form of abdominal ailment (cervical, stomach, colon cancer) place the pack over your belly. For cases such as lung cancer place the pack over your chest. If you have a skin disease place the pack over the affected areas.

Once application is complete, use a warm wet towel to clean the area.

Relationships
We are social beings by nature. The people in your life can make a big difference in your return to health and should be engaged. Often they want to but they just don't know how. Encourage them to read this and to participate with you. If they are part of your household they probably should undertake some of these changes with you.

Sleep
During sleep the body rebuilds itself. It is important to get as much as you need (most people do not get enough sleep). Listen to your body and it will tell you what it needs and when. It is likely that you will need a lot of sleep at first. As you heal your sleep pattern will become normal. If

---

[6] Edgar Cayce is known as the 'Sleeping Prophet'. Check reference section for details.

your sleep is not restful try taking melatonin. Sleep pattern is a great indicator of progress and we will discuss it further in chapter 4.

Exercise

The body is meant to move. Our lifestyle is far from that which our body is designed for. We spend way too much time sitting and indoors, not using our body/muscles as intended. This leads to many issues and affects you physically, mentally and emotionally.

If you are not accustomed to exercise start simple by just walking 30-60 minutes a day. Walk with deliberate focus (no phone, music is OK) and as fast as you can.

If you are too weak to even walk start with simple body movement such as raising your arms, moving your legs and just deliberate breathing. Work you way to walking and to other forms of exercise (like yoga), as you get stronger.

If you can and are strong enough, take yoga classes and do yoga daily for at least 20-30 minutes[7]. You will be amazed at what it will do for you.

If your lifestyle is active (sports, running, cycling, etc.) you should continue to do so regularly and with focus. Do not over stress yourself by working out too hard or too long. During this time of healing you want to avoid taxing yourself.

Routine

During the healing process you should establish a daily routine. This is a time of adjustment, self-reflection and self-care. You will not be partying, staying up late, going out dining, eating ice cream, drinking coffee or doing any of the other things that tend to occupy a day in the life. Your routine will be 100% focused on your wellbeing.

It is OK to engage in relaxing activities such as walking along the beach, going to the movies (no stressful movies, popcorn or any 'movie' food), visiting with friends (as long as they aren't going to engage in stressful activity with you) and anything that is relaxing.

Your Job

If you work you have to assess the impact of your job on your life. Your job can kill you (seriously). Almost half of the people I've helped had to stop working and/or change jobs in order to facilitate healing.

---

[7] Yoga is not really about physical exercise (it is a journey to mental discipline) but is learned through strengthening physical movements (asanas) that are very helpful.

If your work exposes you to any toxins (nail salon, auto paint shop, mechanic, landscaper-excessive sun) or demands a large amount of stress (law enforcement, EMT, emergency room medics) you should consider taking time off or even changing careers.

Any job that exposes you to toxins in any way or is physically demanding is probably a job that you'll have to quit. Your body is ill, meaning that it cannot cope with the exposure that it is getting. It is a sign that you may have to reinvent yourself.

The same goes for any job that causes stress and that you are not enjoying. Some stress is normal and even healthy. But if it wears you down, irritates or depresses you, etc. it is probably not the job for you and your body is telling you so.

The Nice To Do's
Not totally essential (I have seen people heal without these changes) but definitely helpful, these changes are your choice. You may want to try these to see if they are something you wish to adapt.

Meditate
I have meditated most of my life. The ability to quiet the mind and stop thought is so powerful it is difficult to describe. If it didn't require discipline and could be achieved easily I think many people would engage in it.

When you achieve a meditative state you stop thinking. Most people do not know what this is like and will likely never experience it. Quieting this 'little voice in your head'[8] takes you to a place so serene and peaceful that it cannot be described. Once you experience it you want it over and over. It is the true natural high – achievable without drugs or any type of external stimulus. It is our true state of oneness.

But achieving it is a journey. Learning to quiet the mind takes time and practice, usually a minimum of about 6 months if you are really disciplined, to years if you are not[9]. Most people don't stay with the process long enough to get there. I discuss meditation in more detail in chapter 7.

---

[8] For a great read on 'the little voice in your head' read 'The Untethered Soul' by Michael Singer.
[9] My own experience was about a year. It becomes second nature with time. The time frames are based on conversations with others.

Fasting

Fasting is a quick way to detoxify the body. In some parts of the world it is a standard approach to helping the body heal. In the US it is frowned upon. It is not for everyone and if done must be done carefully and correctly. It is an entire process in and of itself. There are many stories of people who attribute regaining their health to fasting. I discuss it in more detail in chapter 3.

Environment

Our 'man-made' environment is filled with toxins. We spend most of our time indoors in artificially ventilated rooms, our days handling man-made objects, and our focus on external gratifications. Most people don't realize how 'unnatural' this is because it is the norm.

If we had more awareness of what works for us (as humans) we could do so much better. Man lives against his nature throughout most of his life. That is why we find nature so rewarding. It is where we are meant to be most of the time yet it is where we are the least of the time.

Disease can be a direct manifestation of environmental stress. If your job exposes you to extremes or chemicals (think nail salons or working in a paint, shop-really bad), your life depends on leaving it.

The same is true in our homes. Most people use toxic cleaners around the house, for laundry and in their yards. You probably bathe with detergent based lotions and bars (which aren't soap). Healing requires change around all of these areas.

Definite Musts

You have to do everything possible to get toxins out of your life. It is amazing how many toxins surround us. For the most part, if it is man-made it is likely to have some level of toxicity.

Our body is made to deal with toxins, as these are a part of daily life even in nature. But modern intervention has created toxins and substances that the body just is not equipped to deal with. It is these (and the excessive amounts of them) that eventually break our body down and cause disease.

Personal

Personal items include anything you use on your person (fragrances, deodorant, soap, shampoo, nail polish, hair color, etc. - everything). You must stop using all products and replace them with the following:

- Shampoo/soap/shaving cream/body wash – Dr. Bronner's pure castile soap. This is an amazing product. Use it to shampoo and bathe, as a hand wash and anywhere you would use soap. It's also great as a shaving cream and has a variety of other uses.
- Hair conditioner/after shave lotion – Organic apple cider vinegar. Mix with purified water 50/50. As a conditioner apply it after shampooing, let it sit for a minute or two, and rinse. As an after-shave lotion dab it on using a cotton applicator. You should leave it on your skin until it dries.
- Toothpaste – Brush with a dab of baking soda. Rinse and then apply 5-6 drops of food grade peroxide to the brush and brush again. Do not rinse. This will do wonders for your teeth and mouth. You will never use toothpaste again (nor will you ever have another cavity). Do not use any kind of mouthwash.
- Deodorant - mineral salt deodorant block.
  Just dampen the block with water and rub on. Rub slowly, 6-8 times per arm.

While you are healing you will not be coloring your hair or using nail polish or any other product other than those listed above. No exceptions.

Household

Most households today are loaded with man-made toxins. Couches, mattresses, cleaners, etc. are all killers. Do a little online research and you will see the poisons lurking in your home and the many issues they are associated with. The same holds true for most household cleaners. As with personal items you must stop using everything and only use the cleaners outlined in chapter 6. Also:

- Ventilate your home – This may be difficult depending on your local weather but try to get as much fresh air into your home as possible. There are a variety of live plants that are very helpful as well[10], if you are so inclined.
- All natural general-purpose cleaners can be found online. Here are a few to get you started:
  - myhealthygreenfamily.com
  - www.apartmenttherapy.com
  - www.keeperofthehome.org
  - www.diynatural.com

You must rid yourself of all cleaners that are not made 100% from the following ingredients:

---

[10] 'How to Grow Fresh Air' by B. C. Wolverton is an excellent resource for plant selection.

- castile soap
- borax
- distilled vinegar
- baking soda
- hydrogen peroxide
- essential oils
- citrus

It is quite easy to use the above to make any household cleaner. Refer to Appendix A for some recipes. I encourage you to do so. There are plenty of online resources to get you started. If you cannot use a 100% organic product do not use any at all. This is important!

- If your home is carpeted do NOT walk barefoot on the carpet. Use natural skin moccasins or flip-flops but do not allow your skin to come in contact with the carpet. Do not sit or lay on it. Carpets are very toxic and let off fumes in addition to collecting dust mites. Using harsh detergents (most carpet cleaners) to clean them makes things even worse. If it is at all possible replace them with ceramic tile or hardwood flooring (not laminate which also has its issues).
- Do not use commercial pesticides. Instead use natural pesticides that you can purchase or make yourself. Some great ingredients are:
  - Garlic
  - Chile pepper (powder)
  - Diatomaceous earth
  - Borax
  - Baking soda
  - Citrus oil

These are just a few of the major areas of the household that must be addressed for healing. Chapter 6 and Appendix C contain more help and references.

1 Why We Get Sick

"The wound is the place where the Light enters you."

Rumi

The human body is amazing, probably the most amazing organism known to man. Millions of cells die and are reborn each day. The body's own hormones are the best painkillers. It is amazingly tolerant to abuse and can adapt to a variety of external circumstances. It can also heal from almost any ailment.

On a mental level, our brain can create 'realities' that do not really exist in our real world. These are so real that our physical body responds to them as if they were actually happening. Our intellectual capacity and self-awareness have allowed us to understand and see the nature of existence and our place in the universe.

Physically we can develop skills and abilities that are so precise that they appear magical. They can make us appear 'super-human' or get us passed physical impediments (such as missing an arm or being blind).

Our body is meant to be in a constant state of balance, known as 'homeostasis'. It has a multitude of mechanisms that all work together to maintain this balance. These respond to everything that happens to us physically or mentally. These capabilities are so powerful that they can cause a state of wellness almost overnight (often called spontaneous remission).

When we fall ill our body is sounding an alarm. Rather than ignore it and attempt to turn it off (this is what is generally

"Our own physical body possesses a wisdom, which we who inhabit the body lack. We give it orders that make no sense."

Jim Rohn

attempted today with medication) the correct response is to understand what the body is saying and take action accordingly so that the body itself turns it off when we get better.

We have attributed a name to almost every form of pain/ailment known to man. Every non-homeostatic condition has a name. And with that

18

name our system of pharmacology wants to provide a way to turn it off. Not to heal it, but to turn it off so we are not bothered by the discomfort this causes. This allows us to continue to function (in most cases) without having to actually address and solve the underlying condition. So when we get a headache or indigestion, we just take medication to make it go away (turn off the alarm) rather than try to understand why we have a headache (or whatever ails us) and address the actual cause.

This process of constantly turning off our body's alarm mechanism and ignoring what we are being told is what leads to chronic disease (which itself is a really loud alarm – emergency!!!!) and eventual death.

First of all, giving every pain/ailment a name and attempting to categorize things and provide categories of treatment (which is what our medical system does today – doctors learn pathology and corresponding pharmacological treatments – nothing about what actually is causing the problem as this is too much work and not economically feasible) is of no value (except to the medical system that profits from it). Every single disease, every one, is caused by one and one reason only; cellular malfunction.

Regardless of what you have been diagnosed with, what is happening in your body is that some group of cells is not working as they should. Restoring them to normal function is all that is needed to restore health (homeostasis). When you are sick this is what the body is trying to do.

Introducing man-made medications will more than likely make things worse. It gives the body additional things to worry about balancing, particularly since many of these substances have chemical makeups that are foreign to what the body is made to handle. That is why natural medicine is safer, the body knows what these substances are and is better able to cope with them.

This isn't always the case. There are some medications that have proven to be helpful to the body. But these are very few. The majority of man-made medical products tend to cause more chaos then good. This is because people are much more complex than their diagnosis. I would venture to say that in many cases people heal in spite of their medications and not because of them.

To attempt to place everyone with a given ailment (i.e. set of symptoms) into the same bucket is one of the biggest problems surrounding modern medical treatment. Every factor in a person's environment affects their homeostatic state. Even good food can be worthless if prepared and consumed incorrectly. The same is true for medication. What worked for one person may not work for another because of all the environmental factors around that person that aren't considered. If the medical establishment took the time to understand each person and what factors contribute to their state of health (on all levels, physical and mental) many more people would be healed[11].

Becoming healthy (achieving homeostasis) is always about understanding what is causing the cellular malfunction and providing the body with the conditions to restore that function to normal. Since each person is different the conditions are always different.

At first glance it seems that this may be something difficult to do. When we look at our lives there are so many aspects to it, habits that we've formed over a lifetime, experiences that make us think certain ways, our likes and dislikes; all of these make up our belief system and everything we do is based on our beliefs.

But two things make the process of achieving health simple; the first is that to make a change in our life all we have to do is change a belief. Once we've done that everything else follows. Our actions automatically mimic our beliefs.

Second is that we have a thorough understanding of the environmental factors that cause imbalance (maybe you don't right now, but you will when you are done with this book). Correcting those factors is actually quite simple as all it takes is going back to what is natural as dictated by our evolution and relation to nature.

Achieving this awareness will allow you to do the things required to bring your body back to a healthy state. And will give you the insight to change your beliefs and avoid the things that cause problems. This is a fundamental understanding and a foundational assumption of this book. It is up to you to do the things required, to listen to your body and understand your 'self'.

It is a great journey. For me it represented a pivotal point in my life, a time when my perspective on everything changed. I learned to live more, love more, and worry less. To listen to and trust my body, to eat right and avoid the many things of modern life that are destructive.

---

[11] Our system, designed for income and profit, does not allow even good doctors to spend the time required with patients to help them.

2 Loving Ourselves and Health

"What happens when people open their hearts?
They get better."
Haruki Murakami

Illness is a cry for help. It is sad that in today's world we use terms such as 'fighting' and 'beating' or 'conquering' our ailments. Do we push away or 'fight' a child when they cry for attention? Disease is our body crying for attention. Warning us that we are neglecting it, not paying attention.

We should see disease in a light of comprehension and growth. It is not a foe to be defeated but a message to be listened to. Your body feeds itself from the source of life. It 'knows' what is missing and what is needed. Healing is paying attention, understanding and taking the required steps to achieve balance. Just as it warns you of imbalances, it will let you know when you are balanced by thriving and being the vehicle via which you live your life.

> "All healing is first a healing of the heart and a cleansing of perception."
> Carl Townsend

Human beings are incredible creatures. We are born with an incredible potential to learn and do many things. Somehow, as we grow, much of that potential goes untapped and eventually many of us become victims of our environment. This leads to the myriad of problems that plague us, from disease and health issues to socio-psychological problems that zap us of our capability to function and live a pleasing and happy life. But if we tap the human potential we can accomplish great things both personally and on a humanitarian basis. Healing is tapping that vast potential.

Many years have passed since the day disease shook my life. My insight into the whys and how has grown considerably. I have discovered that one can live very deliberately, taking very specific actions, and turning life into what we want it to be. And this is true regardless of what adversities might come our way, whether they are big or small, or whether we are blessed with good fortune in any of its many forms.

Turning life into what we want it to be does not mean being able to program and anticipate the events of each day. It is more a way of predisposing

> "When a problem is disturbing you, don't ask, "What should I do about it?" Ask "What part of me is being disturbed by this?". "
>
> Michael Singer

ourselves to events and then turning those that come our way into events that make life worth living. You will see that we are formed by our thought processes in more ways than most people can imagine. Our society as well is the result of collective thoughts and the world itself is in many ways a result of the collective thoughts of humanity.

Being human is indeed a grand and wonderful thing. However it is fraught with mishaps in spite of our capacity to be grand. Due possibly to our relatively rapid evolution we have a tendency towards greed and selfishness. The mishaps and tragic events we encounter are largely a reflection of this greed and selfishness. I've come to believe that

> "It requires more courage to dare to do right than to fear to do wrong."
>
> Abraham Lincoln

underlying these tendencies is something universal to all of us: *fear*. As a matter of fact underlying many human tendencies (particularly

disease) fear sits quietly as a very powerful motivator.

A healthy dose of fear is built into human nature. However as our thinking self has grown more dominant we have developed the capacity to mask it (fear) so well that we fail to see it as foundational to many actions. While fear does have its place it alters the thought process, and subsequently our acts, in unhealthy ways. Once this happens the results are generally devastating to the individual and hence to society and humanity as well.

There is no need to look very far to see how we are destroying ourselves. Despite claiming to be the most intelligent creatures on this planet we are certainly acting like the dumbest in many ways. We cannot seem to coexist with each other. At the world level it is one country/religion/ideal against another. At the individual level it is one neighbor against the other. We speak of love and compassion yet we exercise these only towards those we find are in agreement with our beliefs. We take and we waste resources as if there were no consequences. We take media perspectives for granted and fail to question or understand anything of true relevance to us. Tell me, where is the intelligence in any of these acts?

Healing is largely about becoming the best human being that you can be. Getting there is often a mystery yet at the core of our beings that is what life is about. We are lost... and we want to go home. We want to be great at what we choose to do, loved for who we really are and live each day secure in knowing that our life has meaning and a significant place in the order of things.

Getting to that place of fulfillment should be simple. Our lifestyle often makes it complicated. We are complex beings consisting not only of our physical selves but also of an entire internal universe (emotions, thoughts, spirit) that is at the core of creating our physical manifestation. As we grow and go through life we must integrate these aspects of the self satisfactorily if we are to reach our full potential as humans. In today's difficult, externally influenced world, many of us tend to live shallow lives filled with a lot of meaningless nothings that completely destroy our sense of self. If you are living a seemingly full life yet are frustrated, angry, or somehow feeling incomplete (and continually trying to fulfill that 'emptiness' with jewelry or a new car or by working long hours or by being promiscuous or using drugs or some other form of external gratification) then you are at a crossroad. This moment represents an opportunity to completely change your life and discover for yourself what it means to be happy. Life's measure of success is not in things, what people think about you, or money... it is measured in how much joy you feel each day.

People have forgotten how to be happy. Our societal structure has converted us into victims of external influence. We have forgotten our essence and given up our dreams for material gain and petty pleasures. Indeed, for many the truth is that when you get

> "Wisdom is your perspective on life, your sense of balance, your understanding of how the various parts and principles apply and relate to each other. It embraces judgment, discernment, comprehension; it is a gestalt or oneness, and integrated wholeness."
> Stephen R. Covey

what you think you want you realize it isn't what you want. You probably are working hard going somewhere that in the end you'll realize is not worth going to. It is what society wants you to think you want. There are very many 'successful' unhappy people. If happiness were the goal, our definition of success would take a very different form. Healing is finding the direction that is right for you so that you can reach 'happy'.

In many ways we are always in some process of healing. Most often we think of healing from physical ailments such as cancer or arthritis or some other chronic disease. Or it may be from the mental form of depression or taming some demon that has been haunting us for years. Here I want to focus on how disease happens and how it can be corrected. You will find that disease is intricately connected to the other aspects of the self. Becoming physically sick is usually the final manifestation of imbalances we've been carrying for years. Many diseases are surprisingly simple to reverse once we achieve an understanding of how they become what they are.

Our body is in a constant state of balancing itself against environmental and psychological influences. The key to good health and wellbeing is enabling the body to perform this balancing act. It is a never-ending process that begins when we are conceived and continues until we release our last breath of life. Our goal is to understand what causes imbalances and how to instigate their correction. The rest is accomplished by the miracle of our body.

It is unfortunate that I have to say that relying on society's methods of healing (doctors, hospitals, drugs) is often not very effective[12]. As we go through your healing process you will see why that is true and how you can avoid becoming a victim of the system. The body's capability to heal is immense and should not be underestimated. Yet the medical world is

> If someone is going down the wrong road, he doesn't need motivation to speed him up, he needs education to turn him around.
> Jim Rohn

constantly underestimating this capability to the extent that in most cases it is largely ignored. The input of a qualified physician is helpful but *you* should be establishing the direction of your care as *you* are the one who feels and knows what its like to be you. You should always use this knowledge to better yourself and here we talk about how that can be done. If you are fortunate enough to have a doctor who 'understands' I am sure he will welcome your self-assessment and self-knowledge.

Healing is intricately tied to belief (thus generally begins in the mind). We explore this fact and will learn methods to use it to effectively achieve a state of health. The wonder of all of this is that once you achieve this understanding and align your beliefs your entire life changes in ways that are amazing. It is exciting just to think about the possibilities. As we will

---

[12] Other than the treatment of trauma and surgical processes (which are sometimes required) many patients are subjected to pain and suffering and rarely recover to a state of true health. The medical world's idea of recovery is generally defined as a return to marginal function rather than to homeostasis.

see, healing is an integral part of personal growth. When you heal you grow.

So **Love Yourself**. Start doing the things you've always wanted to do. Yes, there may be (there always are) limitations but that is life. Your intention manifests itself, always. Here are some things you must do:

Pamper Yourself

There are so many forms of self-love that are considered 'special' that really should be part of each day. Start with the simple things:

- Take long hot baths
  You have to bathe regularly so make it yours. Forget the 5-minute shower. Make it an experience. Important pointers:

  o Use only the ingredients recommended in your bath

  o Feel free to add some soft music and candle light (use unscented or essential oil based candles)

  o Focus on breathing and visualizations

- Get a massage
  Touch is an amazingly powerful healing aid. In America it is so under stated and used that it is very sad. If you can, engage in professional massage as part of your healing process. If you have a partner or someone that can give you a massage that is just as effective:

  o Use only essential oil based oil. Use a base of olive or almond oil (if you are not allergic) with a few drops of essential oils

  o If the massage is not professionally administered:

    ▪ Use the palms of your hand

    ▪ Do not cause pain

    ▪ Rub towards the heart

    ▪ Aim for a pleasurable feeling

- Be in nature
  If weather permits spend time outdoors in nature. Sit in the park, walk along the beach, go on a hike, sit by the river, watch the sun rise/set. If weather doesn't allow it sit by a window and watch it rain, or the snowfall, or the wind blow. In short connect with nature.

- Meditate
  Take at least 10 minutes 1 to 5 times per day to quiet your mind. Focus on breathing and not thinking. If you find yourself engaging in thought, direct them to a 'happy' place, a location (real or not) where you are totally at ease and in peace. And focus on breathing, slow, deep breaths.

- Eat Intently
  When you eat, don't be rushed, focus on what you are consuming and visualize it nourishing you. Chew or sip slowly.

Surround Yourself with Goodness

Do not allow for negativity in your life. During healing you should surround yourself with positive people and good thoughts. The people in your life should understand this and support you. Here are some things to help you:

- Laugh
  Watch comedy, read funny books, hang out with anyone that makes you laugh.

- Elicit support
  Tell others how you are working through your condition, what things you are doing. Invite them to try some of your meals. If you have a partner it is important that they play an active role in your support. There will be challenging moments but if dealt with as outlined here they should help you grow.

- Don't complain/criticize
  This may sound odd but is critical. You may have an internal grudge with the world you aren't even aware of. If you find yourself judging or criticizing others put an end to it. Listen to what you say and how you interact with others. Create compassion from within.

- Do what you love
  There is no time like the present to live your life. Learn what you've always wanted to learn. Go places you've always wanted to go.

- Heal relationships
  Do not hold grudges. The effects of a grudge can cause a lot of damage. Reach out to others. Listen more; talk less. Especially to those that are (or should be) close to you.

- Spread Joy
  Smile and say hello to everyone. Be happy. Volunteer[13].

In the end it is about focusing on joy, deciding to be happy. Don't let anyone or anything deter you. Shun negative energy (even if it's your partner, sad is this sounds they may be a part of your illness[14]). Being hooked on happiness is the greatest medicine.

---

[13] Volunteering is one of the most rewarding experiences. Giving freely is helpful to all participants and is needed so badly in today's world.
[14] This is very true. Some of the cases I have worked with came to this understanding and had to let go of 'toxic' relationships.

3   We Are What We Eat

"Life expectancy would grow by leaps and bounds if green vegetables
smelled as good as bacon."
Doug Larson

I don't think there is a person in this country that hasn't heard that they are what they eat.

Eating is something we all take for granted. The great majority of us give very little thought to what we eat other than it must satisfy our immediate hunger. This is only human nature. Not too long ago this is how the body had to work in order to survive. There wasn't a selection of food to choose from. Whatever we could find is what we would eat.

Modern civilization has changed all of that. It is now possible to consume much more food than our body needs with very little effort. The number of choices available is also varied and confusing. As you walk through the aisles of a super market you are presented with hundreds of labels each vying for your attention and selection. Making healthy choices is difficult unless you have a thorough understanding of nutrition and food processing (which probably rules out more than 99.99% of the population from making the best choices).

In addition, modern day food processing has created foods that do not exist in the natural world. This has happened so rapidly that our body has not been able to adapt. This has led to a multitude of nutrition related disorders we see today (obesity, diabetes, high cholesterol, heart disease, arthritis, ... the list goes on; almost every disease can be linked to an environmental influence with food being the most influential[15]). Essentially, today's diet tends to be calorie (and flavor) rich and nutrient poor.

As a result it is important to become aware of what and how much we eat. Doing so is the difference between a healthy life and one that is plagued with health problems. It is sad to say that, in most cases, food related diseases kill the majority of us. Dying of natural causes is a rare thing in our modern world.

---

[15] Today's high incidence of cancer can be readily linked to the increased imbalances created by food. The prolific uses of soy-based products in food, for example, are shown to be particularly harmful and linked to various cancers.

The primary premise (and the singular simplest form of advise I can give) underlying proper nutrition is simple; **avoid processed foods**. This means that anything that no longer looks as it did in nature before you prepare it should be avoided and if it is something that doesn't exist in nature (i.e. soft drinks, pastries and candy) it shouldn't even be considered edible. There are exceptions so I will qualify this as we move forward.

In a world of fast and convenience foods it is no wonder that this is a hard act to follow. It seems that everything in the supermarket comes in a box and is man made. I am hoping to persuade you into spending more time in the produce section of the supermarket where you will find the foods that provide nutritious calories. Consuming these types of foods as the core of your diet is key to optimizing your health.

To be strong and healthy you also have to use supplements. The modern world has destroyed the land's nutrients via fertilization and other mass production methods. Thus most foods are not as nutrient rich as nature had originally intended. There is also substantial research into the use of nutrients that shows how they can enhance body function and slow down the aging process. Add to this our need to constantly adapt to a man made environment that our body is still adapting to and it is quite obvious that the use of supplements makes a difference to our health.

There are hundreds of products out there, some the result of very meticulous research and others just trying to make money. I have spent many years learning, testing and working out the details of what to take and why. You don't have to understand the details (which can be complicated). If you are so inclined the reference section shows you where to go for additional information.

Eating Well

The following sections describe the fundamental eating habits that over the years have proven to be the most effective[16]. Eating habits in today's world are generally based on pleasure and acquired habits that are not in line with how the body processes food. Without trying to be overly monotonous or boring the emphasis here is on eating so that the body functions optimally and food is utilized maximally. Keep in mind that this doesn't mean that eating cannot be enjoyable! There are many good choices of food in most restaurants if you choice wisely. Here are what I consider to be the fundamental rules for eating well.

---

[16] These are generalized indications. While you are ill your diet is much more restricted.

Rule 1: Eat organic

If you are to follow only one of the suggestions outlined here this is it. In all seriousness, modern day agricultural practices are killing you. Many modern farms are no longer farms. They are food mills. Food is produced with a focus on quantity vs. quality. This leads to conditions that are inhumane, unsustainable and detrimental to us all. I cannot emphasize this enough. If you are ill you have likely been a victim of this modern day fiasco.

There is abundant evidence. Appendix C points you in the

> "I would like to see people more aware of where their food comes from. I would like to see small farmers empowered. I feed my daughter almost exclusively organic food."
> Anthony Bourdain

direction of some excellent eye openers and I hope you will use these, and the information I give you here, to become healthy and to support a better way of living. You vote each day with every dollar you spend. If you stop spending on junk and only on quality, the junk will go away and quality becomes the norm. You are in charge and you hold the ticket to a better tomorrow.

Rule 2: Prepare each meal properly

Meal preparation is important as it serves to facilitate digestion. In essence, proper meal preparation can be considered the first step in the digestion process. Proper preparation is simple and can be done by anyone.

Here are the basic guidelines regarding the preparation of meals:

- Start meal preparation with quality food that has minimal to no processing.

- Minimize fruit consumption (humans are NOT natural fruit eaters) and do not combine fruit with any other food type (i.e. eat fruit alone).

- Be careful about combining food types.

- Aid digestion with proper preparation.

The above guidelines are probably counter to what many of us do when we sit down to eat. This is part of the reason why most people have food related problems (often without realizing it) and why in most cases food is digested poorly.

The body utilizes different enzymes to break down food based on the type of food being consumed. These enzymes have different characteristics and may not work together well, particularly when some are acid and others are alkaline. The combination of these enzymes causes their effectiveness to be reduced and thus the digestive process is compromised. Often this produces gas, bowel irritation and other discomforts (including acid reflux/heartburn). This is a stress that, over time can cause severe problems[17].

Does this mean that the good life of food indulgence is over? For many of us eating large, diverse meals with lots of flavor is a great pleasure. The key word here is *pleasure*. There is nothing wrong with a properly prepared grand four-course meal. As a matter of fact I know an excellent cook that prepares great meals consisting of a variety of items each served separately yet in a complimentary fashion. Her meals are appealing, delicious and nutritious[18].

But on a regular basis our eating habits should be simple and governed by the rule of minimal combining. This isn't as bad or difficult as it sounds. It's just a matter of acquiring some basic understanding. It is also conductive to simple preparation that hopefully makes it easier to fit the meals into hectic schedules. As you heal you should learn to make eating this way a part of your daily life.

Rule 3: Eat more early and less in the evening

Again, this is contrary to how most people eat. You should have your biggest meals during breakfast and lunch. Dinner should be very light and no later than 2 hours before going to bed. Yet in today's world dinner tends to be the biggest (and worse) meal of the day. Just adapting this practice will help you lose more weight than many of the popular diet plans being used today.

The logic is simple; ingest more calories when your body is using them. Starting each day off with a large breakfast will actually make you less hungry and more energetic throughout the day. Likewise eating less later in the day is conducive to better rest and sleep at night.

---

[17] Be warned that most medical doctors disagree with this. Note that most medical doctors know very little about nutrition and are themselves victims of these issues.
[18] Follow the links in Appendix C or the recipes in Appendix A for great meals.

Rule 4: Snack well

It is good practice to have light snacks between meals. A good snack helps curb appetite and keeps your energy levels stable. The key here is that it must be a good snack and it should be kept light. A good snack is fiber rich and minimally processed (almonds and walnuts are a good example).

How to combine food

The general idea behind combining (or not combining) food is based on how the body digests different food types. Some foods are minimally digested when combined with other foods. This leads to reduced nutrition and often, to various degrees of discomfort and indigestion. If you exhibit any of the following symptoms after eating you are doing something wrong:

- Abdominal discomfort/indigestion

- Heartburn

- Gas

- Headaches

- Runny nose

If you eat a typical meal it is likely that afterwards you will feel bloated, tired, gassy and overall just lethargic. You have effectively filled your body with food that complicates digestion due to the way its been combined. Each type of food requires different enzymes to digest. While your body does a pretty good job at producing these their effectiveness is reduced when they get all mixed up (similar to how watered down juice loses its flavor). So much of what you eat goes undigested. It reaches your colon in a state where it proceeds to wreak havoc, causing you to feel lethargic and eventually making you sick.

Now, your doctor will likely tell you that this is all nonsense. Do a search and you will come across the 'debunking' theories (and it's all they are is theories). They'll bombard you with all sorts of scientific reasons why this isn't so[19]. My suggestion to you is to experiment and try for yourself. If you observe carefully you will develop a keen sense of how food (and food combining) affects your body. I've become so good at it that I can spot it in others even though they have no clue what is happening. I really wish advice were more factual than theoretical (and we were open more to learning). Whenever you come across this type of controversy first ask the advisor if his knowledge is practical or theoretical (most doctors are theoretical – until they get sick themselves; the wise ones wake up, others become victims of their own methods... sad). Then take some time to explore yourself. It only takes a few meals to see what is happening[20]. Anyone that has actually taken the time to explore and understand will tell you it makes a major difference.

> "In theory, there is no difference between theory and practice. But, in practice, there is."
> Yogi Berra

Now before we all get paranoid this doesn't mean that our body can't handle combined foods, just not as effectively. The pancreas (as all body organs) is amazing and can produce all sorts of enzymes concurrently. Some foods do combine well (some combinations do taste great!) and some should freely be combined as desired. But what can and can't be combined does matter. You give your body less stress and better absorption capability when you combine wisely, especially while you are ill and healing.

This is critical. Even consuming all the right food in the wrong way will cause problems. And the typical diet, the way you've probably been eating most of your life, is just a major problem. There are many resources on the Internet. Listen to your body! The following guidelines should help achieve better eating habits with increased nutritional benefits.

- Always eat fruit alone (and only 1-2 times per week)! As a general rule, minimize the amount of fruit you eat (1-2 times per week) and eat fruit on an empty stomach. Fruit can be divided into four groups (i.e. as in a fruit salad). These are:

---

[19] I contend that with everything we think we know about the body we still know very little.
[20] There is an approach to doing this called the 'food elimination' diet. It is based on starting with a very clean set of foods and slowly adding foods to learn how they affect you.

- o Melons
  Always eat melons by themselves. Melons do not digest well when consumed with anything else.

- o Citrus/acid
  Oranges, grapefruit, tangerines, strawberries, pineapples

- o Sub acid
  Apple, Papaya, Peach, Pear, Raspberry, Apricot, Blackberry, Blueberry, Grape, Cherry, Mango, Guava

- o Sweet fruit
  Bananas, Dates, Figs

Try not to mix fruit across groups. Mixing them within their own groups offers the best nutritional value and ease of digestion.

- Proteins require the strongest digestive enzymes/acids. Once the body starts digesting protein other foods will largely go undigested and will reduce the digestibility of proteins. This will lead to fermentation in the colon that can lead to many health problems. Passing gas often is a sign of colon fermentation. Thus it is best to consume proteins without combining with other food or combined with green leafy vegetables or legumes.

- Carbohydrates are a flexible food. Properly combined they offer very nutritious options and very complete meals. I generally combine carbohydrates as follows:

  - o Raw vegetables
    These are the typical components of salads and include leafy greens and other vegetables that are consumed raw.

  - o Cooked vegetables
    These include legumes and vegetables that are generally cooked.

  - o Grains and starches
    Our body is not good at digesting grains and starches[21]. Due their abundance these have become staple food for

---

[21] Humans have only been consuming grains since the advent of agriculture. Our bodies have not evolved to handle this kind of food.

many. Consume only small amounts and only whole grains. Grains generally digest better when combined with legumes.

- In general raw vegetables are digested slightly differently from cooked vegetables. Refer to the reference in Appendix A for details.

- Avoid the consumption of cold liquids. Any cold liquid (even water) inhibits digestion. Liquids should be consumed at room temperature (between 65 and 72 degrees Fahrenheit).

Calories and weight

Food consumption for diets is generally measured in calories and divided into protein, fat and carbohydrates. This is a modern day misconception that assumes that calories and weight are directly related. Not so. While there is a relation between calories and weight it is not a direct correlation. Eat the right foods as outlined here (larger meals early, small meals late), consume the right kind of foods (minimal preparation, non man-made) and you will be consuming food that is in line with your needs and will allow you to lose or gain weight without the need to count calories and check portion sizes.

Here is a simple pointer; if you want to lose weight just stop eating all forms of grains, starches and fruit. Stick with proteins and vegetables and you will lose weight rapidly and without starving. Start your day with a high protein breakfast[22] and just watch the weight melt off.

While you are healing these guidelines will be a little different to address the healing process. The particular foods you consume or the portions are what you adjust. You still apply the guidelines in every way possible (i.e. avoid processed or man made foods).

These are the basic rules of eating well. If you stick to these you will change your life and your health dramatically for the better. Weight balance will happen naturally and you won't have to starve yourself or do anything out of the norm.

Here is a typical day of food for me as an example:

- Upon rising I mix 1 tbsp. of apple cider vinegar with a cup of water and the juice of one lemon.

---

[22] Tim Ferris (4 Hour Body – see references) did great research on this. He coined the term '30 in 30' meaning 30 grams of protein within 30 minutes of awakening.

- Within about 15 minutes I consume a protein/vegetable drink made of fresh vegetables and natural protein (from peas and rice) in water[23].

- Mid morning snack: nuts (usually almonds, walnuts and peanuts). Sometimes I add dried cranberries.

- Lunch: Legumes (beans or lentils) w/4-5 oz. of ocean fish (or organic pork) and steamed vegetables

- Mid afternoon snack: nuts and coffee or green tea

- Dinner: 4 oz. sardines with steamed vegetables

- Bedtime: (same as rising) mix 1 tbsp. of apple cider vinegar with a cup of water and the juice of one lemon

That's a basic day. Note that while you are healing your food consumption will be much more restricted and limited to what is outlined in 'Immediate Actions' at the beginning of the book. Once you are healed you can begin to eat a larger variety of food. Sometimes (maybe once every 2 weeks) I'll enjoy things like ice cream or cake (I love chocolate). I tend to have one or two glasses of wine per week.

This is just an example of an eating pattern that abides by the rules stated above. You should make up your own based on your needs and preferences, taking care to be true to yourself. Once you are healed and recovered, eating pleasurable foods (dessert, wine, etc.) is OK as long as it is done with moderation.

Supplements

Many of today's foods are depleted of vital nutrients. This is a sad side effect of mass production and inadequate rebuilding of soil. As a result much of the food we consume is not as rich in nutrients as it should be. Therefore it is important to supplement the diet with concentrated nutrients.

Our need for certain nutrients changes as we age. Therefore I've divided the recommended supplements into two groups; base nutrients and over forty. Again, while you are healing you will abide by the instructions

---

[23] Consuming protein early in the day helps regulate insulin and appetite throughout the day.

provided at the start of the book (Immediate Actions). When you are well follow the supplement schedule outlined here (which is very similar).

Base Nutrients

There is a basic nutritional requirement for all adults that we should all meet. Even a good diet won't provide you these nutrients in amounts that are really beneficial, particularly if you are ill. The table below outlines the supplements that you should take. Appendix A provides dosage and brands.

Supplement	A M	P M	Why
ALA-ALC	X	X	Promotes cellular function. Required by all cells. Promotes cellular energy metabolism. Memory boost.
Flax oil	X		Provides essential fatty acids
Omega 3-6-9		X	Provides essential fatty acids
Sulfur (MSM)	X	X	Synergist to EFAs. Multiple body functions.
Coenzyme Q10	X		Heart/circulation, immunity, Multiple body functions.
Coenzyme B Complex	X	X	Essential B complex. Coenzyme is better used.
Chromium polynicotinate	X	X	Insulin stabilizer. Retains and supports muscle tissue construction. Improved body mass.
Selenomethionine		X	Anti-oxidant, immune booster
Zinc picolinate		X	Metabolic enhancer, Immune booster, male health, reproductive health
Ester C	X	X	Anti-oxidant, immune booster
Vitamin D3	X		Skin/bone health, helps mineral absorption

Over 40 Nutrients

Supplement	A M	P M	Why
DHEA	X	X	Important hormone regulator/stimulator, immunity booster, insulin regulator
Melatonin		X	Sleep regulator, anti-oxidant, mood enhancer
Pygeum/Saw-	X	X	For males only. Male health.

palmetto			
Glucosamine/Cho ndroitin	X	X	Joint/Bone health.
Calcium/Magnesiu m	X	X	Joint/Bone health. Metabolism. Mental support.

In general, the body starts to age at around 35 years. This means that around this time tissues start to degenerate and organ function begins to diminish. There is extensive evidence (myself included) that demonstrates that proper care and use of the body will retain function for extended years (I am 55 and just as strong today as I was when I was 35 – I still wear the same size as well).

Edible Food

You can eat as much as you want... as long as you eat only food from the lists that follow. It is that simple. As previously mentioned most of today's foods are, in one form or another, of little to no value to you or worse.

Modern day convenience is probably one of the major diseases we suffer from. However, convenience is not classified as a disease (how convenient). Due to convenience we pay crazy prices for water in bottles (not to mention the environmental damage to aquifers), single use cups (which are also toxic), items wrapped in plastic that we just remove and discard, 'preserved' food and all sorts of other 'convenience items'. Instead of cooking fresh food we buy packaged food that is so far removed from its source that its nutritional value is dubious at best and its preservative content is guaranteed to be beyond anything we should be ingesting. But shelf life is increased and life is so much easier! Convenience is killing us. I consider it a disease in everyone I've helped.

So let's be clear. Learn to prepare your own food, eat food at locations that prepare it well, or continue the path of illness with its inevitable consequence. Look around you for anyone who has died of natural causes. In the USA you'll be hard pressed to find someone because in today's world everyone is expected to die sick. And be assured that the system will finish you off with its numbing medication while getting every last possible dollar out of you while you're on your deathbed. And they'll make it look like they care.

I apologize for my moment of digression. I hope it is clear how I feel about convenience and food. Feel free to research and investigate for yourself. There is plenty of evidence. It is only a matter of time before we regress back to a more effective way of life (the digital era and the internet will create awareness to the 'tipping point'). You are reading my contribution to the cause. Through your health and healing you will 'see' and learn for yourself the value of living within human nature. Please spread the word.

Buy Local

In macrobiotics food is classified based on the energy it gives off (Yin or Yang). It proposes that our body is exposed to energy variations from our environment and that food localized to that same environment is best suited to nurture our body.

There are reasons why this makes sense. It is difficult to prove as not much research has been done along these lines. However, based on the fact that this is how we ate for thousands of years (modern technology now allows food to be transported almost anywhere) and that local food is guaranteed to be fresher, it makes sense to eat locally as much as possible.

I suggest finding a local farmer's market and taking advantage of it. The prices are great and the produce is fresh and in season. It is not always organic so be careful. And farmer's markets tend to be a nicer trip than going to the supermarket.

Vegetables/Greens

Our body has been designed through many years of evolution to obtain its nourishment from the greens around us. Nothing will change that. Therefore the bulk of what you eat should come from organic vegetables. They should be consumed raw as much as possible and cooked carefully when cooked. Here is a list of common vegetables you should consume (ordered alphabetically, non-exhaustive):

Vegetable
Artichoke
Arugula
Asparagus
  Green, Purple, White
Avocado
Bamboo Shoots
Beet
Bell Pepper
Bok Choy/Bok Choi/Pak Choy
Broccoli
Brussels Sprouts
Burdock Root/Gobo
Cabbage (green/Red)
Capers
Carrot

Cassava/Yuca
Cauliflower
Celery
Celery Root/Celeriac
Chayote
Chinese Broccoli/Kai-lan
Corn
Cucumbers
Daikon Radish
Eggplant
Endive
Fennel
Horseradish
Kale
Kohlrabi
Leeks
Lemongrass
Lettuce
Lotus Root
Lotus Seed
Mushrooms- see Mushroom List
Napa Cabbage
Okra
Olive
Onion
Parsley
Parsley Root
Parsnip
Peppers
Plantain
Potato
Pumpkin
Purslane
Radicchio
Radish
Rutabaga
Sea Vegetables:
    Arame
    Hijiki
    Nori
    Wakame
Spinach
Squash- see Squash List
Sweet Potato
Swiss Chard
Tomato
Turnip
Water Chestnut
Water Spinach
Watercress
Yams
Zucchini

This is perhaps the most neglected of the food sources, yet it is one of the most nourishing. Legumes are amazingly nutritious. Essentially, they are the seeds of legumes. Nuts are the seeds of trees and are very similar. Seeds generally come from flowers. In their sprouting state they are much easier to digest and are alkaline forming.

If you are ill I strongly suggest you sprout legumes for consumption. It is actually quite simple and will provide great benefits, mostly digestive. Here is a short list of legumes to choose from:

Legume	Cooking
Beans Adzuki Black Soy Red Pinto Kidney Lima	Beans must be softened (overnight) or sprouted (about 3 days) before consumption. See Appendix A for details. Beans can be combined with seaweed (arame or hijiki) for greater nutritional value. Try one of the recipes in Appendix A.
Peas	Peas vary in how they are cooked depending on the type of pea. See Appendix A for details.
Lentils	Lentils do not require softening and can be cooked in under 30 minutes. Sprouted lentils, like beans, are easier to digest.
Nuts (raw) Almonds Brazil Cashews Hazelnuts Pistachios Pecans Walnuts	Nuts should be eaten raw and unsalted. Eat them daily in small quantities as a healthy snack. A few nuts go a long way. Do not grind nuts (or purchase them ground) until they are ready to consume. Notice the absence of peanuts. Peanuts can be very toxic and should be avoided.
Seeds Flax Chia Hemp Pumpkin Sesame Sunflower	Seeds generally come from flowers. The seeds outlined here are what I consider the most valuable. It is best to grind the seeds when they are ready to be consumed. See Appendix A for ways to include seeds in your diet.

Animal Proteins

As omnivores our body is designed to consume animal protein. In today's modern world there are a variety of reasons why consuming animal protein may not be the best choice. But it isn't because they are bad for us. It is because of what modern day agriculture has done to meet this consumerist demand that has led to the sad state of affairs surrounding our food sources. Much more can be done to produce food properly and with respect for the animals and our environment.

Be sure to purchase all animal protein from a reputable source. The handling of animal proteins makes the difference between healthy and toxic.

We consume much more animal protein than we should. In general, 3-5oz per serving is more than enough. Yet on average we consider protein the primary ingredient in most meals. This is not healthy for us or for our environment. I suggest consuming the majority of protein from non-animal sources (legumes) and supplementing it with no more than one portion of animal protein per day.

Having said that we'll consider the value of animal protein to our health.

Ocean fish is possibly the safest protein left to us in today's world of artificially produced (and processed) animal foods. If you are going to consume animal protein then seafood protein is the healthiest bet. Of all seafood, my all time favorite is the sardine.

I know many people do not like sardines (I see the looks on faces when I devour them). However, sardines are amazingly rich in many essential nutrients. I tend to consume whole canned sardines in water or olive oil at least twice a week.

Generally most ocean fish are healthy and you should consume some form (4-5oz. is enough) a few times each week.

Shellfish can be healthy but this is dependent on where it comes from. Generally, cold-water shellfish is of higher quality than that from warmer water. If you are ill DO NOT consume any type of shellfish. If you do consume shellfish be sure of its quality.

Chicken is probably the most consumed of all animal proteins. Naturally raised, organic chicken is a good source of protein. The problem is that most chicken isn't. Do not consume any chicken that is not labeled as organic and hormone free. It is in your best interest.

Eggs are very nutrient rich. They should come from organic sources as well. Contrary to popular belief, eggs do not cause high cholesterol[24]. The combination of any rich source of fat with unhealthy sugar (i.e. starchy food and fruit) is proving to be the trigger for formation of LDL cholesterol. During my athletic years I consumed 3-6 eggs daily and my cholesterol was always around 140 (90-50, I have hereditary low LDL).

---

[24] Cholesterol is still highly misunderstood. There is strong evidence that high cholesterol levels are induced mostly by sugar rich diets that ingest saturated fats.

Red meat, when proceeding from a natural source is also very healthy. I consume venison when I find it at the farmer's market. Venison is around 8% fat versus 35% fat for supermarket red meat. Meats such as veal are worse (not to mention the inhumane animal treatment) and should never be consumed. Consume only organic, naturally raised red meat or do not consume any at all.

Of all animal proteins pork is perhaps the most nutritious and digestible. However pork production is also highly hormone rich and inhumane. It is difficult to find good pork from an organic, naturally raised source. If you can find a quality source then consuming pork a few times per week is a healthy choice. But probably 90% of the population does not have access to the quality required.

Given the problems surrounding animal protein production my suggestion is to stick to vegetable proteins (see Appendix A) and limit animal protein intake to seafood unless you happen to run into organic sources.

Herbs

The power and value of herbs is highly underestimated. Today most herbs are used for flavor. Herbs do so much more and that is a good thing.

Cooking Herbs

Herb	Uses/Benefits
Basil	Anti-bacterial, anti-inflammatory
Cilantro	Antioxidant, metal cleanse/detox
Cinnamon* (1/2 tsp)	Antioxidant, anti-inflammatory, insulin facilitator/anti-diabetic, anti-bacterial
Cumin* (1 tsp)	Digestion, diabetes, weight loss
Fennel	Anemia, stomach issues, menstrual issues
Garlic	Detoxifier, anti-inflammatory, anti-infection
Ginger	Digestion, anti-inflammatory
Nutmeg	Digestion, sleep, skincare, brain health
Oregano	Anti-bacterial, anti-oxidant
Parsley	Anti-oxidant, heart, arthritis
Rosemary	Memory, mood, pain relief, stomach, anti-bacterial
Saffron	Anti-depressant, eyesight, memory
Sage	Anti-oxidant, anti-inflammatory, memory
Thyme	Anti-oxidant, anti-bacterial
Turmeric	Anti-inflammatory, arthritis, cystic fibrosis

Tea Herbs

Herb	Uses
Chamomile	Anti-bacterial, stomach, sleep
Echinacea	Anti-oxidant, anti-inflammatory,respiratory issues, painkiller
Green tea	Anti-oxidant, brain health, weight control
Ginseng	Weight control, sexual health
Lavender	Digestion, relaxant/anxiety, anti-fungal/bacterial
Milk Thistle	Liver, skin
Peppermint	Digestion, anti-microbial
Rosemary	Brain/memory, anti-bacterial, anti-oxidant

Liquids

Modern day liquids are key contributors to the destruction of health. Everywhere you go what is offered, no matter what you choose, is bad for you. Essentially, if it comes in a container it is bad for you. What you read on the label of these containers is mostly marketing nonsense, created by ignorance and hoping to feed on ignorance.

Basically the only liquids that are good for you are water that you filter yourself, teas that you make yourself, green juices that you make yourself and fruit juices that you make yourself (on occasion).

For example, any fruit or vegetable juice sold has to be pasteurized (heat treated), a process that destroys and changes the characteristics of the juice, essentially killing it. Mostly, what is delivered are useless sugars. There is no such thing as a prepackaged juice that is good for you. Period.

But it's big business, so there are many companies out there trying to convince you that these products are nutritious and good for you. Again, you vote with your dollars. And if you purchase this stuff there will be more to sell.

Bottled water is perhaps the biggest rip off of all time. Anything bottled in plastic, regardless of what it is, has toxins that you consume when you drink from it. Studies[25] have yet to find a plastic that is safe and non-toxic for food consumption.

One case that I worked with had cracked, dried lips. She had tried all sorts of balms and prescribed ointments with no change. On the surface she seemed to be doing everything right. She ate organic, took care in meal preparation, etc. One day she casually mentioned to me that

---

[25] A quick internet search will show results and conclusions. Thebest studies are mostly outside the US.

44

buying bottled water was getting expensive. Alarm!!!!!!! I hadn't realized she purchased and drank bottled water exclusively. I told her to stop, filter her water and use a stainless water container to drink water from when she was out and about. In less than 2 months her lips were totally recovered.

Not every case is so extreme but it shows the impact that toxicity in plastics can have. Plastics have done some great things for our modern world. But using them as food containers is not one of them. Stay way.

Many food items can actually be made more digestible by 'pre-digesting' them as liquids. This is the general idea behind smoothies and juicing. The idea is a good one and generally nutrients in liquid form are easier to consume and provide more nourishment. The key is to make sure the right ingredients are combined.

The recipes in Appendix A will show you how to prepare liquids that are good for you from wholesome ingredients. They are simple to prepare and will nourish you.

Fruit

Most health journals and articles will lead you to believe that fruit is wonderful and good for you. Well, sorry to break it to you but fruit, while it does have great nutritious qualities, is generally not good for you.

History shows that fruit is not a natural part of the human diet. Our body really doesn't know how to digest fruit. Research has been done that shows the effect of fruit on the body the moment it is consumed. Insulin spikes, glucose storms, pancreatic craziness, it all happens within minutes of that first bite. Some research I have done leads me to believe that some people die of fruit related dietary problems without even knowing it.

This doesn't mean you shouldn't eat fruit, only that you should limit fruit intake to no more than 2 times per week, and consume it alone as a snack. Some fruit, lemon in particular, affects the body in a different way. I suggest lemon use regularly as outlined in Appendix A.

Grains

Grains are right up there with fruit. Grains are the seeds of grasses. Our body generally has no idea what to do with grains (or starchy food in general). Grains were never part of the human diet until the advent of agriculture so they've only been a part of the human diet for about 10 thousand years (which is nothing in terms of evolution). They are popular because they are easy to grow in abundance and convenient (did I mention convenience is a disease?).

When you do consume grains organic whole grains are the best. Like their relatives the legumes, sprouted grains are also easier to digest. Some of the recipes in Appendix A use grains and provide further details around their preparation and consumption.

All the rest

If it is not mentioned here it is because I don't even consider it food and neither should you. This includes dairy products, man made goodies (cookies, cakes, etc.) and the like. Does this mean that we should never eat these things? The short is answer is absolutely not while you are sick and healing and very (and I mean very) moderately when you are well.

The world seems to have an obsession with dairy products. Our body naturally reacts to dairy products negatively. We are so accustomed to these effects (sneezing, runny nose, gas, mild indigestion, lose stool) that we do not realize that dairy could be a major cause. I distinctly recall the sense of wellness that I started feeling just days after I stopped using dairy products.

It's OK (as long as you're not ill) to have the occasional ice cream or milk shake, or to enjoy a little bit of cheese with wine. But to use dairy products regularly will lead to long-term issues.

I love chocolate (and cookies/pastries in general). I will have some here and there but very sporadically. Since everything is OK my body can deal with the stress and I can enjoy the treat. By sporadically I mean like once a month, maybe.

I am also a coffee drinker. I drink coffee or green tea almost daily. Coffee has a variety of benefits and as long as it is not abused should be OK for you. Drink your coffee earlier in the day. I tend to have mine mid-morning and mid-afternoon. Do not exceed 40oz. per day and make sure it is quality coffee, not decaffeinated (decaffeination introduces toxins) and fresh brewed.

Fasting

Fasting is controversial, mostly because it is so misunderstood. The fact is that fasting helps the body by giving it a break from processing food and allowing it to cleanse and clear the digestive tract.

I go on 24-hour fasts regularly, about once every 5-8 weeks. During this time I just drink water and green tea.

More extended fasting is helpful, especially if there is a lot of toxicity and excessive weight. I have read cases of fasting as long as 60 days!

How does one fast for that long without starving? Well, the answer is that when you fast you still nourish yourself. You use very rich vegetable broths and/or melons (there is such a thing as a water melon fast). I do not recommend fasting for longer than 3 days without supervision, as it is important to understand what you are doing.

If you are ill try fasting one day a week. During this day drink plenty of water and make a vegetable broth by combining 5 or more vegetables with water, bringing them to a boil then simmering for about 20 minutes. Consume only the broth. Consume hot green tea as well.

When we are ill our body will often tell us to fast by not inducing hunger. Listen to this call. During this time drink water and rich vegetable broth as mentioned above. Your body will thank you for it.

4   Taking Back Your Life

"To insure good health: eat lightly, breathe deeply, live moderately,
cultivate cheerfulness, and maintain an interest in life."
William Londen

Whenever we think of 'me' we generally see ourselves as physical
beings. As we go through life we learn to connect to the world around us
mostly on a physical level. This is normal as we are physical beings from
the day we are born until the day we die. We learn to feel, see, hear,
smell and taste and as we associate these sensations to the resulting
experiences they bring us we label them good, bad, indifferent or
somewhere in between. As we gain more of these experiences we start
to direct our actions in ways that help us achieve the sensory
experiences that we have marked as good and avoid the ones marked
as bad. Time brings us new sensations and thus our memory of good
and bad grows along with our arsenal of actions to achieve those
(sensations) we like or avoid those we don't like.

In essence the above paragraph summarizes how we learn to live.
Basically most of our behaviors are geared towards achieving sensations
that we consider pleasurable. These range from simple things like eating
or taking a warm shower to the thrill of going on a white water rafting trip
through the Grand Canyon. We also develop protective behaviors to
avoid 'bad' things such as being yelled at by our parents or losing our
jobs. But in reality it isn't losing our job that we are avoiding. It is the
resulting 'bad' things like not being able to eat at our favorite restaurant
or losing our comfortable apartment and its resulting pleasures that we
are avoiding.

If we analyze this process further we realize that we are acting out of
fear; the fear of not being able to achieve those good sensations or of
experiencing 'bad' ones. Think about this for a moment. Fear guides
many actions. It is important to understand this in order to embark on this
journey of personal growth.

Returning to physical sensations, it is possible via physical activities to
reduce the stress that comes from the activities that we endure in the
quest for what pleases us. Let us begin with the most fundamental needs
and learn what is essential to our physical selves.

Basic Needs

As the human fetus grows (before birth) its needs evolve around the development of the physical and sensory system that eventually propels us through our physical existence. The first sense to develop during this process is the sense of touch. All other senses are derived from the core nerve system that begins with this one sensation. As a newborn, touch is essential to proper sensory development. Without it, even if every other need is met, the newborn will die.

Despite the fact that we are not generally conscious of the importance of touch we constantly refer to it in our daily conversation. People are 'abrasive'; we get 'in touch' with each other, some are 'softies' while others are 'prickly' or 'thick skinned'. Sometimes we are 'out of touch' or 'tacky'. The word 'touch' itself is used in ways that allude to pleasantry; someone has 'a professional touch' or a 'soft touch'. A nice gesture is considered 'touching'. When we are attracted to someone we want to touch them or they 'touch' our heart. As children we have a natural tendency to touch and openly express the need to be touched.

Bring us to adulthood. As adults most of us are touch deprived. We rarely come into close contact with each other. While some of us have the good fortune to be surrounded by huggers (my personal circle of friends is very touchy-feely) most people do not receive enough tactile stimulation to be healthy. The symptoms of this are readily visible and also readily ignored. They range from common symptoms like headaches to more severe nervous disorders. The sad thing is that so few people are aware that the cause for these is touch deprivation that they go through life in a form of tolerance and reluctant acceptance (or worse, they use drugs or sex to numb the discomfort). Physical wellbeing is not possible without touch.

Another area that causes many subtle (and sometimes not so subtle) problems is breathing. While we all take breathing for granted the grand majority of people breathe in very shallow patterns that deprive the body of full oxygenation. The consequences of this shallow breathing are again often ignored. Normal breathing is overlooked and underemphasized. Have you ever heard a doctor say that you have to improve your breathing?

Our body is attuned to our breathing patterns. Just hyperventilate for a minute and you will see how it completely changes how you feel. Or take slow, deep breaths for a few minutes. You will immediately see the effects of breathing on your body, not to mention your mind. Breathing patterns establish a rhythm throughout your body. It is as if your body is an orchestra and breathing is the conductor. Many body functions can be regulated by the conscious and methodical use of breath. This is a large component of a technique called 'bio feedback'.

Effective breathing is directly related to effective brain function. Most people enjoy going to the ocean. While there are many reasons for this one of the reasons often cited is fresh air. One of the outcomes of being close to the ocean is often a higher mental acuity and inspiration. Many great thoughts and epiphanies happen while we are walking on the beach. These things happen for various reasons one of which is the quality of the air and a tendency to breath consciously when we are close to the ocean. Finally, conscious breathing provides focus.

Our next basic need is that of nourishment. I include here not only our need for food but also our need for water. While this area gets a lot of attention most of the data is irrelevant to what really matters (much of it is market/profit driven fad). There are so many miracle diets out there that it is impossible to amass them all into one publication. The benefits of these are dubious in many circumstances and non-existent in others. The bottom line regarding nourishment is simple: keep it simple (as outlined in chapter 3), the simpler the better.

Body movement (or the lack of it) is another major cause of problems. More than 90% of people do not get enough exercise to maintain a healthy muscular/skeletal system. The big excuse is usually a lack of time. Yet the ailments produced by lack of physical activity take more time from us than if we invested some time in productive exercise. Our body is designed to move and not doing so is a major cause of problems. Aging and loss of muscular and skeletal tissue is greatly accelerated by lack of physical exertion.

As our society has grown and become more (and more) 'unfit' the standards for being fit have been continually lowered. If we use a fair fitness standard to assess fitness more than 95% of the population would not be fit. And what is even sadder is that most people don't realize the benefits of physical fitness. Quality of life and productivity increase dramatically when the body is in a good state of fitness.

Many years ago, while on a weekend cycling trip, I met an older fellow cyclist. On the second day of riding we were offered two possible bike routes. One was beautiful, scenic and strenuous and the other was plain, easier and shorter for the less experienced riders. I asked Alex about his plans and he said to me he didn't have a choice, for him it was the easy route. I had grown fond of our conversations and was tempted to accompany him on the easy route. He turned to me and said, "You need to take the scenic route because you can. I started too late and my body has never been strong enough but yours is and you can so you should".

As we talked later that day (I did take the more challenging scenic route) I learned that he took up exercise at a late stage in life. He was happy he did but he was sad that he hadn't done so earlier and now realized how much he missed out on just because he had been out of shape.

Don't let this happen to you. There are many things you can enjoy in good fitness that you cannot if you are not fit. And we will see that being fit, while it does require commitment and discipline, does not take much time at all. Now is the best time to start.

There is a significant amount of talk about the benefits of exercise and numerous books, programs, clinics, etc. Yet the majority of people still don't do so. We will discuss the possible true reasons for this (lack of time is not one of them) throughout this book and will address them.

Last but not least is Rest. In today's fast paced world very few of us get the rest we need. Here I want to point out the importance of adequate rest and how to fit it into our daily life. Without adequate rest many of our body functions are impaired, leading to a multitude of stress related disorders.

We have to build a method of taking care of our physical self that encompasses and maximizes the benefits of these five areas. They work together to build and maintain a body that serves as the foundation for a better life, just as a good foundation is the prerequisite of a well built building. Without a good physical foundation there are limitations to how much of our human potential we can achieve.

Furthermore, the methods and activities that result from this foundation should fit into your life as an integral part of it, not as some additional activity that you have to make time for. Proper living is an accumulation of acts and habits that make up your life in such a way as to facilitate achieving your goals in a stress free, humane and positive way. Let us explore each area in detail.

Touch

Many of you will find it hard to believe this but if you can improve only one aspect of the physical self the most beneficial improvement is likely to be in the area of touch. Just being hugged and hugging another person 4 times a day will foster great improvements in physical well being. Add to that a weekly massage and your physical health will start to improve dramatically almost instantly.

I find it curious that in the medical world the power of touch is largely ignored. As a matter of fact, most MDs have virtually zero understanding of the myoskeletal structure and its contribution to overall wellbeing. Chiropractors and touch therapists (massage therapists, acupuncturists, structural integrators) are the exception as their methods of healing require the use of touch and they are familiar with its benefits.

Here are some facts about touch that you are probably unaware of:

- Skin is the largest organ in the body and represents between 15-20% of body weight

- All of our senses are developed from tactile nerves while in the womb

- 90% of nerve endings are connected to the skin. There are over 5 million of these

- Every one of the nerve passages of the body (there are 12 – called meridians) ends in the hands and feet

- Any form of pain can be reduced by touching the skin

- Touching the skin produces oxytocin, a feel good hormone

- Touch improves mental acuity

- Touch heightens other senses

In numerous studies, research has found that the power of touch is capable of healing physical and mental disorders. As a matter of fact touch has proven to be effective in the treatment of practically all ailments.

Touch largely gives us our sense of reality. Anything you can see or envision in the physical world is in some manner associated to touch. Objects are solid, or hot or soft or tangible or intangible. Many blind people develop a sense of touch so acute it is like 'seeing' through the skin.

I hope this gives you an understanding and awareness of touch and its importance. Awareness is a key first step towards incorporating the right acts into your life.

Incorporating touch into one's life should be a natural occurrence. Here are some possible ways to bring touch into your life without changing anything except the way you feel:

- When speaking or watching television with someone we trust make skin contact

- When speaking with colleagues it should be normal to tap each other on the shoulder, make hand contact ('hi fives' or hand shakes) and other such gestures

- On a more intimate level, partners should massage and rub each other every day.

   o A five minute back rub before going to bed or upon awaking or while watching television should be part of daily communication

   o It costs absolutely nothing to rub your partner's feet or hands while watching a movie

   o Provide a 2 minute shoulder rub while he/she is doing dishes

   o Try a facial massage using only your finger tips

   o Shampoo each others' hair and rub the scalp deliberately for a minute or two while lathering and while rinsing

These simple acts of touch improve relationships and the overall well being of those involved:

- Hug each other! Learn to hug on hello and goodbye even among men

- This is difficult in many of today's cultures as such gestures have been misconstrued with ridiculous taboos and implied meaning. I don't expect that many of you will do this but one can hope.

- Get regular (weekly is ideal) massages, acupuncture, reflexology and the like. Alternate between methods. While this can be a bit expensive you can reduce the costs by locating schools where students need to practice. If you are older than 50 the costs will more than likely be less than the alternative medical costs you would require. It is too bad that insurance companies and the medical community don't understand this. You will come to agree that the benefits outweigh the costs. If you are a couple or a family you can learn to massage each other by going to a workshop, using videos and/or reading. This will cut costs and provide many benefits.

- Scrub your skin while bathing. Bath gloves or Japanese bath towels are an excellent way to do this. They offer the additional benefit of skin exfoliation (removal of dead cells and dirt) in addition to excellent stimulation. When using bath gloves apply soap to the gloves themselves then use the gloves to lather yourself up. When rinsing first rinse your bath gloves (while wearing them) then use them as you rinse the soap off of your body.

- Many of us have difficulty reaching our backs when we bathe. This tends to cause hygienic neglect. The large skin area of the back is also a great area for stimulation. I have found two effective ways of reaching the back while bathing. You can use a back scrubbing shower brush or, and this is my favorite method, you can use a Japanese bath towel. These can be found at Asian grocery stores or on the Internet (see resources in Appendix C). Once you try one of these you will be hooked!

- Stimulate your ears with bath gloves or a hand towel. Ears are very sensitive. Stand under the shower with water running down the back of your head. Use bath-gloved hands to stimulate your ears by rubbing and pinching them. When done right this will usually send shivers down your spine. Oh what a feeling!

Doing any of these simple things stimulates the body by producing hormones that regulate many other body functions. This is the grand benefit of touch. By touching the skin you are touching every part of the body and affecting it in (positive) ways that are still mostly scientifically unrecognized but intuitively understood.

Our physical body houses the tensions and stresses of our daily life. While we often think of things such as anger or fear as mental, when repressed they are housed in our physical body. Touch facilitates the release of these 'accumulated tensions', thus allowing us to relax and be in touch with more pleasurable feelings. Herein lies its power. This is why in a moment of need we instinctively know to hold each other. The comfort and security offered by touch immediately triggers the biochemical release of substances that cause positive effects and allow us to cope with stressing external circumstances in a good way.

It should be simple to make these actions a part of your daily life. This is a crucial first step towards reaching your potential. It will make you feel better and will help you to better cope with life's daily challenges. I've never known anyone that didn't feel better after a good massage, back or foot rub!

Breathing
The first thing we do when we come into this world is inhale and the last thing we do when we leave it is exhale. We can only live without breath for a few minutes, making breathing the most essential of all body functions. Yet most of us breathe incorrectly.

The general breathing pattern of the average person tends to be based on inhaling with the stomach and exhaling with the chest. This method of breathing is both shallow and incomplete, leading to shortness of breath, inadequate consumption of oxygen and minimal removal of toxins.

But why do we breathe this way? The truth is that when we are born we breathe deeply and with our diaphragm (just watch any healthy child under 6 years old). As we grow up and begin to respond to stress this pattern tends to change, becomes shallow, hurried and restricted. Since this happens slowly over many years we adapt and it becomes 'normal'.

Our entire body rhythm is regulated by our breathing pattern. It serves as the orchestrator to many other body functions and patterns. Most of us are in a constant struggle for harmony and aren't even aware of it. Here are a few indications that you are likely to be breathing incorrectly:

- Do you often feel 'bad' or uncomfortable without understanding why?

- Do you inflate your chest when you take a deep breath?

- Do you get mild headaches often?

- Do you feel tense?

- Do you sigh often?

- When relaxed do you take more than 10 breathes per minute?

These are all symptoms of improper breathing. Depending on the severity of your 'bad' breathing pattern you may have other symptoms that can be traced back to breathing. The simplest way to become aware of these is to pay attention to the changes that will occur as you start breathing consciously.

Incorporating proper breathing into your life is a matter of practice. Since you are breathing continuously there are plenty of opportunities to improve and the adaptation of proper breathing is quick.

Breathing is also the foundation of a deeper consciousness. In parts 2 and 3 we use breathing techniques as the gateway to a quiet mind and the experience of bliss. But by far the most notable effect of good breathing will be in physical wellbeing. Here are some immediate benefits of proper breathing:

- An immediate sense of relaxation

- Heightened alertness and focus

- More energy

- Physical problems and pain will lessen (and disappear!)

- Other unexplained symptoms will disappear

- Better sleep

The best part is that the effects of proper breathing are immediate. There are many ways of improving breathing and many different techniques and exercises. However, we will focus on simple, readily adaptable methods that you can practice almost anywhere.

We can look at breathing as a multi step process. We start with simple breathing patterns that teach us how to breathe properly. We can then proceed with more complex breathing patterns aimed at expanding our consciousness and maximizing our use of oxygen.

Lets focus on making you aware of your breathing and learning how to control it. Usually we are unaware of our breathing. This causes us to acquire bad habits (the body has a tendency to be lazy). Becoming aware allows us to change those habits to the point where we significantly improve our unconscious breathing pattern as well.

You can do this while at work, when driving and stopped at a traffic light, while waiting for the bus, as soon as you wake or before going to bed, or at any other moment when you have a few minutes to pay attention to your breath.

All breathing exercises start with proper posture. If you are seated sit straight with both feet flat on the ground and if you are standing stand straight with your weight evenly distributed to your feet. Your shoulders should be level and slightly held back without causing any undue tension.

Now take notice of your breathing. Notice the speed, the depth. Is your chest expanding or are you breathing into your stomach? Is it silent or can you hear yourself breath?

Now place your hand on your tummy. Start breathing such that your tummy is now expanding and contracting as you breath. Your chest should not expand but should move naturally as a result of your tummy's expansion and contraction. Become fully aware of breathing in this manner.

As you exhale squeeze slightly to make sure you exhale completely. As you inhale try to slow down your breathing but make the inhalation more complete by absorbing more air into your tummy.

Follow your breath for a few minutes while keeping your attention on this pattern. Notice that your mind will probably wander and you will forget that you are focusing on your breath. Whenever this happens and you become aware of it just return to your breathing pattern.

It is good to become accustomed to breathing this way. In particular it is good to do this whenever you are not feeling well (headaches, in pain, sad), nervous or just in need of a few minutes of relaxation and stress relief.

Expansive Breathing

The body is meant to breathe effectively while in motion. Expansive breathing is about fully expanding and contracting our ribcages while offering a very effective stretch. This is a good way to start your day when you get out of bed:

1. Start by standing with your feet slightly further than shoulder width apart. Keep your shoulders back but relaxed and look straight ahead of you. Finding a focal point at eye level is helpful.

2. As you inhale raise both arms straight in front of you, synchronized with your inhalation. While continuing to inhale, bring both arms around behind your back and clasp your hands at the highest point that you are able to without bending your elbows. Look upward while completing the inhalation and consciously expanding your rib cage.

3. Hold this position for about 5 seconds and also hold your breath during this time.

4. With your chest still expanded and arms still back behind you (elbows straight) begin to bend forward at the waist while slowly beginning to exhale. You may bend your knees slightly as you bend over as far as is comfortable for you. With time you should be able to get pretty far without bending your knees. Your exhalation should be synchronized with your movement such that you will complete exhaling by the time you are bent over as far as you are capable. Hold this position for about 2 seconds making sure to exhale completely.

5. As you begin to inhale start bringing yourself up to a standing position. As you complete standing unclasp your hands and let them settle at your side while completing a deep inhalation.

6. Exhale slowly, focusing on a full exhalation and releasing any tension you have in your body. On your next inhalation begin the entire movement again.

You should repeat this movement about 5 times. It is a good morning stretch to perform when you get out of bed (see chapter 5). I also like to do this movement (once or twice) in the middle of the day when I need a good stretch and reenergizing.

Practicing these two breathing methods regularly will do wonders for your breathing pattern and overall wellbeing. The key is persistence. It is easy to find moments each day when you can focus on breathing.

Whenever you have an idle moment you can consciously breathe. It will make a big difference in your life.

A very practical way to improve your breathing, overall fitness and mental focus is by practicing yoga or martial arts. These are both excellent disciplines with many benefits. In both cases breathing is at the center. It is possible to integrate yoga into your life within the time spaces you already have in your day.

To learn more about breathing, techniques and approaches used by others you can refer to any of the resources in the Appendix C. The Internet has many good resources, there are workshops and of course there are various good books that focus solely on the subject of breathing.

Relationships

We are social beings. It is well accepted that without meaningful relationships life itself is meaningless and unhealthy. At the root of many illnesses we find loneliness, a lack of meaningful connection to others. Not making oneself known to another human being is a self-imposed sentence of misery and pain.

Life is all about relationships. From our first relationship with our mother we spend our entire lives surrounding ourselves by relationships. We make friends, we have business relationships, we get married, and we have children. Look at the popularity of social media (Facebook, twitter, SMS, etc.) and you'll see that life revolves around our relationships.

It takes being true to oneself to see within and understand what our relationships (or lack of) mean to us. On the surface we all want to tell ourselves that we have great friends and partners. But to really know a friend or be intimate with a partner requires that we remove the façade and truly see what is there. Fear of confronting our aloneness is worse than confronting it.

Some of the greatest research done on relationships clearly shows that when relationships are good among people life flourishes in amazing and gratifying ways. We are more productive, healthier, compassionate and empathic. It is easy to say that happiness equals good relationships.

When relationships are not good, on the other hand, life becomes painful. We seek refuge in drugs, alcohol, promiscuity; we look for ways to numb the empty feeling. Eventually, this kills us, bringing on disease and the mental and physical breakdown of our bodies.

It is important, if you are ill, to look at your relationships and understand how they may be playing a part in your illness. Illness may happen in spite of good relationships but it is important to know that the stresses of emptiness are not contributing or affecting it negatively and are manifest physically.

What makes a good relationship? When a relationship is good we know so intuitively. It feels right. Just the thought of that person brings a sense of goodness, inner peace and strength to us. One strong relationship is more effective than 100 shallow ones.

Likewise, if we are surrounded by shallow relationships that are manipulative, relationships where we are trying to get something out of each other, then our relationships become toxic and troublesome. Consequently we become unhappy and eventually sick.

We can say that a good relationship in any aspect of our life is:

- Sincere, compassionate and empathic.

- Accepting and non-manipulative.

- About listening and understanding or speaking empathically.

- Cooperative. What binds you makes you a team.

- Supportive. Making each other better people.

For relationships to work you must be your own best friend. You must **ALWAYS** love yourself first. Take time to understand who you are and become your own source of joy. You will have more to share with others and others will have more to share with you. No one makes you happy. You make yourself happy and you share that with others.

Happiness
Life is about joy and happiness. It is so important that the pursuit of happiness is alongside life and liberty in the US constitution. Yet in today's hectic world it seems so hard to find happiness.

Yet happiness is a choice. It is the choice we make as to how to respond to the circumstances we face each day. It is quieting the little voice in your head that is constantly telling you what is right and what is wrong. If you allow life to unfold and learn to follow its pattern you begin to see that the pattern is always inclined towards what you want manifest, to what you desire. Your thought patterns have much to do with happiness.

So think good thoughts. Laugh, dance, sing[26], don't worry be happy. Here are a few pointers:

- Don't take things too seriously
  Worrying about anything you can't control is wasteful and harmful. Take a deep breath and let it go.

- Who cares what others think/say
  Someone will always be there to criticize something. The truth is that as long as you are doing what gives you joy and are not hurting or degrading anyone life is good.

- Do what you want to do
  As long as you treat others fairly follow your own path. Create your own rules. Make your life yours. Who says things have to be a certain way?

Remember that your life is yours. Happiness is your choice. Adversity is always opportunity. Make it count.

Fearlessness

As stated earlier, fear tends to govern many aspects of our lives. Most change is about letting go of fear. The fear of failing, for example, keeps many people from doing things they would like to do.

Overcoming fear is mostly a mental adjustment. Fear stems from our capability to see the possibilities of an act before they occur. Those possibilities are based on our experience until that moment.

For example, some people love water. They see water and they just want to dive in, go sailing, etc. Others are afraid of water. They only want to be as far from it as possible. When you trace these two paths you find a different set of life experiences.

Those who love water associate it with positive experiences; refreshing, abundance, the breeze, etc. Those who fear water may only remember the time they almost drowned, or how cold it was the first time they

---

[26] Studies show that humming has a beneficial effect on health and attitude.

jumped in. We tend to see each moment in our lives based on what we've experienced. Those things we anticipate as good we embrace and those that we believe will result in a 'negative' experience or avoided. That is fear.

If you are ill, it is likely that your illness is creating a lot of fear. If history shows poor success rates (as with cancer) the fear can be overwhelming, making matters more difficult to correct.

Society has done illness a great injustice. It is often referred to with terms such as monsters and evil, the enemy, something we fight and beat. This creates many of those fear-filled images for those that have disease.

Imagine, on the other hand, that illness was seen as an opportunity to grow, something to embrace and teach us to live better lives. Then, when we got sick, we would look at it with a different perspective and would treat it in a different way.

Well, disease is just that, our body telling us, in its infinite wisdom, that something is wrong and that we must learn what it is and change it.

Each fear in life is faced with a choice; we can succumb to fear and not take action, become its victim, missing out on whatever experience overcoming it would bring. Or we can look it in the eye, understand it, and go beyond it. Here are some thoughts on working through fear:

- Embrace it
  The first step in getting passed fear is to accept that it is there and embrace it.

- Understand it
  Take time to understand what precisely makes you afraid.

- Research/Read
  Learn about what you are afraid of. It will open your mind to new perspectives and possibilities.

- Release control
  Don't try to control it. Accept what is before you and learn from it.

- What is the cost?
  What happens if you don't act? If you do? If you fail? Oftentimes we make things much bigger than they really are.

- Visualize
  Visualize success. In detail. See it, feel it, hear it, smell it, taste it.

Other practices suggested in this book, such as meditation, will also help. In the end an overall approach to changing your life for the better will reduce your fears.

5 Moving For Health

"Those who think they have no time for exercise will sooner or later
have to find time for illness."
Edward Stanley

I don't think there is anyone reading this who hasn't heard about the importance of exercise. So I am not going to say it again (at least I'll try not to). What I want to do is offer alternatives that you can incorporate into your life that will not be any more disruptive than you would like, provide you advice to make sure you exercise correctly and point you in the right direction if you want more information. Physical exercise must be incorporated into your life just as food is.

The body becomes sick from not moving. It is not meant to not move. If you are ill learning to move your body, as it needs to be moved, will help you heal.

To be fully healthy, the body needs three forms of physical movement. In some cases it is possible to combine these whereas in the majority of cases they are addressed separately. It is entirely up to you how you choose to incorporate these into your lifestyle.

The first form of movement is stretching. The role of stretching in fitness is supplemental. It prepares the body for functional movement and facilitates recovery from functional movement. It is more therapeutic with a role of integration and balance.

We instinctively start each day by stretching. Notice when you get out of bed how you will tend to yawn and stretch as you begin to go about your day. It is your body's way of aligning itself after lying immobile through the night. I am going to suggest that you extend that morning moment with a simple stretching routine that will do wonders for your body.

As we go through life our body adapts itself to the environment we expose it to. Physically, it adjusts itself to perform our repetitive daily physical activities in the most efficient way possible. Thus it adapts itself to how you walk, stand, sit, the things you do repeatedly and any other physical habits that you have (such as carrying a purse or walking in heels).

While this may sound wonderful it is actually the source of many problems. You see, the activities that we subject our body to are often 'unnatural' and are rarely done while our joints our perfectly balanced. This causes our basic body structure to become unbalanced as it adapts to the task at hand. As time goes on this becomes a part of what is called our 'soma'. This causes problems that are termed as 'structural'. These problems cause many aches and pains and in very severe cases will disrupt our ability to function and in all cases limit our capacity to function efficiently. Proper stretching helps counter the effects of this 'structural disintegration', enabling us to function more effectively and with much less physical pain.

The second form of exercise is what is called endurance or aerobic exercise. It is particularly beneficial in improving heart function, circulation and the efficient use of oxygen. It is very effective at burning fat. Reducing fat and improving oxygen uptake are key to optimum health. Our body is designed to function aerobically (as in chasing prey or running from danger). The problem is that in our modern society this function is no longer really needed. This causes physical degeneration.

While it may not be our goal to be endurance athletes it is our goal to improve our aerobic function so that we are healthy. Examples of aerobic exercise include brisk walking, jogging, cycling, swimming, aerobic sessions at the gym and a few other not so common forms such as weight training circuits and vigorous dancing. Essentially anything that raises your heart rate above around 110-120 beats per minute (this is an approximation as it is age dependent and varies from person to person) and keeps it there for at least 15 minutes can be considered aerobic exercise.

The third form of exercise required is strength building exercise. Its primary benefits are increased strength, improved bone density, more muscle mass, improved tone (this keeps your body in the right position(s) when you are sitting, standing and relaxing) and improved metabolism.

The most popular form of strength building exercise is weight training. But there are other forms that are also effective including freehand resistance exercises (like push ups), the use of bands for resistance and even agonist-antagonist resistance movements.

Exercise is essential to healing as it helps normalize the body. During exercise the body responds with the production of bio-chemical reactions that make it function more effectively. Follow the guidelines at the beginning of the book to adapt exercise to your recovery. After you are healthy you may consider adapting some of the practices outlined here.

Our goal here is not to become exercise gurus or body builders or Olympic athletes but to achieve a balance between life and a commitment to exercise that will allow us to live more effectively, the definition of 'effectively' being that we are not prone to any of the diseases that come from bodily misuse or lack of its use. This is accomplished by an adjustment in lifestyle that will include exercise, not as a 'chore' but as an integral part of living. I will provide guidelines but it is up to you to choose the activities to incorporate into your life. If you are ill, follow the guidelines at the start of the book in 'Immediate Actions'.

It is important to start with a benchmark. Therefore we will start by first assessing where you are in terms of health vs. where you should be. This is dependent on gender, age, height and weight. Within your category you will be guided through a series of activities. The result of these activities will be compared to an accepted standard. Our goal will be to either get you up to the standard or to keep you there if you happen to already be there.

If you are young you can build and sustain your condition well into your older years as long as you don't lose it. While it is never too late to start it is better to start early and make good life habits a part of your lifestyle. I am 55 years old as of this writing and I can outperform almost anyone half my age!

Assessing Readiness
Before even starting you have an idea of your overall state of health. If you do not have any medical or physical ailments and you are not visually overweight then it is likely that you are ready to start executing the exercise programs outlined in this section. If you are not exercising regularly start VERY slow and allow your body to build itself up. If you are uncertain as to your ability or at what exercise level you should start consult your doctor, preferably one that understands exercise physiology

(seriously, this is not funny but many doctors know very little about fitness[27]).

If you already exercise regularly then you can feel confidant that using these programs as a guide to adjust or vary your lifestyle will be simple and will enhance your position. However, I do want to point out that while many people claim to exercise regularly many do not do so correctly. This is, in my opinion, a major cause for concern as improper exercise can worsen your overall health and/or cause injury. You cannot just decide to start running, put on a pair of running shoes, and go to it. There are correct ways to run, breath and build up without causing an imbalance. While at the gym I see many people just walking around from exercise to exercise without any structure or proper execution form. This is very bad! I have worked with many cases of tendonitis, fasciitis and other conditions all caused by improper exercise execution. So please be careful.

Be realistic in assessing your level of fitness. When was the last time you ran over 50 yards? How many pushups can you do without straining? If you are not fit and athletic, start SLOWLY. Do not overestimate your fitness level.

Stretching/core building

Stretching can be incorporated into a day of activities very easily. I suggest that you start each day with the simple stretching/breathing sequence below. Following that sequence is a set of stretches that should be performed at various points throughout the day. The key is to develop the habit of stretching. If you pay attention to your body you will learn to know when a stretch is necessary. As you begin to feel the effects of stretching you will more readily know when to stretch.

Performing a stretch properly is extremely important! Pay close attention to each description. Video sequences for each movement are available on the website and should be viewed until you are sure that the movement is being performed as required.

If you are a yoga practitioner and have a regular practice (which should be daily and no less than 3 times per week) then you are more than likely already performing an adequate stretching sequence and can continue

---

[27] At one physical checkup the doctor wanted to send me to a cardiologist because my heart rate was too slow!!!! I'm an endurance athlete where resting heart rates under 50 bpm are typical.

with that. Read through the following paragraphs and use your best judgment on how to proceed.

Morning stretch/breathe sequence

It is suggested that this sequence be performed daily upon awakening. It is excellent in bringing about full alertness and balancing the body after a night's sleep. It also helps build core strength and muscle tone.

You will notice that there is a very specific breathing pattern for all of the movements. Breathing is a part of everything we do and is integrated into each of the descriptions. It is important to pay attention to, and breathe properly.

Expansive Breathing
This is the same breathing sequence outlined in chapter 4. Use it as the first movement of your morning stretch.

Standing warrior
This is a variation on a popular yoga pose. It is designed to build strength and tone the entire body while stretching the shoulders and torso. You should go into this movement directly after completing expansive breathing.

1. Start by inhaling and bringing your arms up and touching your middle fingers behind your head with elbows pulled back while looking straight ahead and slightly up.

2. As you exhale bend your knees and begin to squat, stopping after about a quarter squat. Hold this position and complete the exhalation.

3. While holding this position inhale slowly and deeply into your abdomen. Exhale and continue to hold the position. On your next inhalation straighten your arms overhead and, in one continuous motion, lower them until they are pointing straight ahead in front of you. Hold this position for 5 breaths. If you are having difficulty sustaining the pose for the 5 breaths you may keep your legs straighter so as to reduce the effort or you may do less breaths and work your way up to 5.

4. On your last exhalation return to a standing position and bring your arms back to your sides.

Torso arching (Cat-Cow pose)

This is a popular yoga pose. It is simple yet effective at producing spinal freedom and toning the muscles of the torso.

1.   Bring yourself to the floor on hands and knees. Do so by squatting, leaning slightly forward and placing your hands in front of you about shoulder width apart as your knees come down to the floor.

2.   Continue moving your body forward until you are resting on your hands and knees. Your arms and upper legs should be perpendicular to the floor.

3.   As you inhale arch your back while raising your head towards the sky, creating an exaggerated arch with your torso as you look up. Hold for about 5 seconds.

4.   As you begin to exhale reverse the arch (in rhythm with your breath) so that your back is now completely hunched as you look towards your navel and complete the exhalation. Hold for about 5 seconds.

5.   Repeat steps 3 and 4 for a total of 5 complete breathing cycles.

Cyclist's Bend

This movement is an excellent balance builder and strengthens the back and core muscles.

1.   As you complete the prior movement (torso arching) sit on your heels while keeping your feet straight on the floor. Place your hands behind your head with fingers intertwined.

2.   While you exhale raise your buttocks off your heels slightly (about 3-6 inches) and bend forward, arching your back, bringing your face as close to the floor as you can without losing balance (and falling forward). As your core strength builds you will eventually be able to bring your face within an inch or two of the floor but you shouldn't rush this. Perform the movement very slowly. It should take you between 6 to 10 seconds to completely exhale and bring your face close to the floor.

3.   As you begin to inhale bring yourself back to the starting position. Focus on straightening your back one vertebra at a time. Again,

move slowly, taking between 6 to 10 seconds to complete the inhalation and movement.

4. At the top of the movement (and the completion of your inhalation) pull your elbows back with your upper back muscles.

5. Repeat the movement slowly 5 times in complete synchronization with your breath. Remember to take at least 6 seconds to go down and another 6 seconds to come back up.

Abdominal compression
This movement focuses on your core and toning your abdominal and frontal (pushing) muscles.

1. At the completion of the Cyclist's bend place your hands on the floor on either side of you, roll back on your hips and thrust your legs forward so that you end up sitting on the floor with your legs stretched out in front of you.

2. On your next exhalation fall back slowly so that you are lying on the floor with your arms at your sides. Inhale.

3. As you exhale raise your torso and legs simultaneously, keeping your arms parallel to the floor until your arms cross your knees. Complete your exhalation and hold this position for a moment (about 2 seconds).

4. As you inhale slowly bring down your torso and legs until you are lying on the floor again.

5. Repeat the movement slowly 5 times in synchronization with your breathing.

At the completion of the last movement remain lying on the floor and focus on your breathing. Visually see your entire body relaxing, working your way up from your toes through your feet, legs, your back, chest, left arm, right arm all the way to your face. Try not to think about anything. If you find your thoughts wandering return to focus on your breathing. Listen to your heartbeat and feel the sense of calm that permeates through your body as you rest. You should continue this breathing/thought process for about 5-10 minutes if time allows.

When you are ready you should rise slowly with the help of your arms. If you have back problems roll over onto your side and bend your knees, rising onto them before bringing yourself up to a standing position. You may feel like stretching again. Take a deep breath and stretch your arms overhead.

You should strive to do this sequence of movements daily. It is a great way to start each day. Within a few days you will notice how much better you will feel and how much stronger you are getting. Strengthening your core and proper breathing will go a long way towards improving your overall wellbeing.

Find a pleasing location to do this. If you are fortunate enough to be able to do this outdoors, perhaps looking out over a garden, the woods or the ocean, you should do so. If you are limited to doing it in your hotel room (as I often am) open the curtains and let natural light in. The idea is that your surrounding should be as pleasant as you can make it. Busy places like the gym are not good locations. Having said that, do the best you can with what you have but be sure to do the sequence!

Stretching throughout the day

As you go throughout your day it is important to keep your physical body limber. The body was not meant to sit at a desk in front of a computer for hours on end, or to stand behind a counter or even be subjected to continual un-symmetric movement (i.e. construction work, walking around a retail store rearranging merchandise, performing patient tests in a hospital, slouching on the couch while watching television, etc.). All of these things contribute to altering/creating your somatic pattern and adapting your body to positions and movements that cause it to lose its integral structure. In essence, our daily activities have a tendency to alter our body in a manner that is not conductive to good health over the long term.

Stretching throughout the day counters this effect and will do wonders to keep your body properly aligned and structured. The following suggestions should be taken seriously and made a part of every day. They don't interfere with your day and will help keep you strong and pain free for many years.

Seated Stretches

Most people spend a large part of their day seated in front of a computer and/or behind an office desk. Many also spend between one to two hours each day sitting in a car, train or bus. Our bodies were not designed for long periods of seating and adapt negatively to this (lack of) activity. The side effects of this are many. Some common ones include back discomfort, shoulder problems, carpel tunnel syndrome, de-toning of musculoskeletal structures and loss of bone density just to name a few.

But this need not be the case. The following suggestions will do wonders to avoid these conditions and many others and will contribute to better posture and increased mental alertness. All you have to do is just do them!

Before we get to the stretches per se a word about the proper way of sitting is in order. You are seated properly when your back is in its straight, relaxed position and your torso's weight is distributed evenly on your hips. Maintaining this position should not require any effort on your part.

To sit in this manner your feet have to be flat on the floor and your knees should be comfortably bent at a ninety-degree angle. For any length of sitting of more than five minutes this should be the norm. Crossing your legs, slouching or any other unbalanced form will lead to discomfort and body issues over the long term.

So why is it that sometimes crossing our legs or slouching feels comfortable? The short of it is that the body needs to move regularly while seated. Muscles become 'tired' of being idle. So it feels good to change your position. Proper stretching takes care of this need in a way that does not have detrimental side effects. It allows you to sit properly for long periods thus keeping your overall body structure in better balance. Over time this can be the difference between having and not having back, neck or knee issues. We spend a lot of time sitting down so it should be done properly.

Seated overhead reach
This is a simple movement that should be done at least every 45 minutes of sitting or more frequently (pay attention to your body and you will know when).

1. Start by sitting up straight in your seat and placing your feet flat on the floor.

2. Take one or two slow, deep, breaths as explained previously. When you are ready, inhale and clasp your hands (fingers laced) behind your head. Pull your elbows back gently as you complete the inhalation. Hold this position for a few seconds.

3. Proceed to straighten your arms overhead and apply a mild tension to your shoulders as you try to reach towards the sky.

4. With your arms still overhead add a slight side bend to each side, feeling the stretch down to your waist.

Seated leg stretch
This is another simple movement that should be done at least every 45 minutes of sitting or as needed. It is designed to be done while seated so you don't have to leave your desk.

1. Start, as always by taking a couple of slow, deep breaths as discussed previously. Be sure to sit straight with both feet flat on the floor.

2. Begin by extending one leg out in front of you (usually under your desk) and hold it flexed for a few seconds before bringing it back down to the floor. Repeat with the opposing leg and repeat two or three times with each leg.

3. Now flex one leg, taking your foot off the floor, and grab it at the ankle, pulling it up for a good stretch. Repeat with the opposing leg.

These two stretches are all that I do while seated for long periods. There are variations and I'm sure you can think up a stretch or two so feel free to experiment. The key here is to stretch regularly so as to keep the body happy and free of burdening patterns.

It is always good to move while working. Try not to spend too much time in awkward, unnatural and unbalanced positions. I getup often for water and bathroom breaks and, if weather permits, go outside for a breath of fresh air often. It is a matter of making these things habit and understanding that staying in any one position for longer than a few minutes is not good for you and should be avoided by stretching and moving.

If, on the other hand, your job requires constant motion (woodworking, store clerk, cashier, gardener, etc.) you should be careful to move without undue strain. Each job has its own potential issues. Try to make the best assessment of yours. Listen to your body.

Endurance
Endurance is probably the area of exercise that is most ignored. While it is not difficult it takes time to incorporate endurance exercise into our daily lives. Yet endurance is the most important form of exercise for keeping your cardiovascular system working optimally (and avoiding

heart disease and other forms of circulatory diseases, some of the nation's biggest health problems).

The good thing about endurance exercise is that it can, and should be, fun. An hour 3-4 days each week of racquetball, tennis, basketball, cycling, dance aerobics, swimming or other aerobic exercise (or a combination of these) will keep your cardiovascular health in optimum condition for an entire lifetime.

More, of course, won't hurt. If you love to play basketball just play all you want. The key is to spread it out fairly evenly over the course of a week and combine it with a good warm-up while avoiding excessive strain. It is not good to concentrate 4 hours of basketball, or any other aerobic activity, into a Saturday morning each week. This is counter-productive and will eventually hurt you.

As an example a good week of endurance exercise would consist of an hour of cycling on Monday, a dance aerobics class on Tuesday, racquetball on Thursday and perhaps a two-hour bike ride on Saturday. The key here is that the activity is evenly spread over the course of the week. Of course, you should build a schedule that fits into your life but you MUST do so.

If you are out of shape, ill, and/or over weight you will have to start slowly. A good start is to walk as briskly as you can every day for 30-45 minutes until you are in good enough shape to practice full blown aerobic activities. If you do take up walking you should walk as fast as you can. A leisurely walk may feel relaxing but is NOT an aerobic activity.

So what can be considered an aerobic activity? In brief it is any activity that will elevate your heart rate to where your heart is exerting itself at least at 65% of its maximum capability and held there for at least 20 minutes. Your heart's capacity varies with age, fitness level and genetics but the following formula will serve as a general guide:

$(220 - age) * .65$

This formula will give you a general idea of what your minimal heart rate per minute should be to be within your aerobic range. This is a generic formula. The only way to determine your exact range is to run a physiological aerobic test under strict conditions. How this is done is beyond the scope of this book but if you wish to learn more please refer to the reference section.

To keep track of your heart rate you can measure your pulse (the poor man's way) or you can purchase a heart rate monitor that will constantly monitor your rate while you exercise. This is a very worthwhile investment. You can obtain one for as little as US $50.

If you decide to use the poor man's way here is the process:

1. Start your aerobic activity.

2. After you reach your expected sustained level of effort (usually after about 10-15 minutes) use your index and middle fingers to find your pulse on your neck right next to your Adam's apple.

3. Using a watch with a second hand, count the number of pulses for 15 seconds.

4. Multiply by 4 and this will give you your approximate heart rate per minute.

You should repeat this at least twice during your aerobic activity to make sure you are working hard enough. Generally, if you are working hard enough you will be sweating and cannot sustain a continuous conversation.

Which brings me to my next point. Be sure to drink water at least every 15 minutes during your aerobic activity. It is best if the water is not cold as this allows you to drink more water and is more in line with your core body temperature. You should drink about 4 ounces of water for each 15 minutes of activity, more if you feel the need to do so.

My final point is about breathing. Be aware of your breathing and breathe deeply and into your tummy. Try to breathe through your nose. If you are gasping for breath and breathing through your mouth you are very likely over exerting yourself.

If you are practicing a rhythmic aerobic activity such as running, cycling, swimming, climbing a stair master or elliptical machine, your breathing and your pace should be synchronized. Focus on your breathing and exercise form until you find a pace that feels comfortable (but still is causing you to keep your heart rate at or above the aerobic level).

More Advanced Technique

If you are fit and want to try more advanced work you can try maximization sprints. This type of activity can be cut down to about 30 minutes and is very beneficial. Basically, a maximization sprint is a very intense effort sustained for a minute followed by a minute of rest and then repeated. You continue in this manner for at least 10 cycles. The intensity of effort will do wonders for increasing your endurance, performance and cardiovascular fitness.

Say, for example, that your chosen activity is running. You start by warming up for about 10 minutes with an easy jog. At this point you do your first sprint. For 1 minute (timed, accuracy matters here) you run as fast as you can without being reckless with your form. Immediately after the minute you slow down to an easy jog (or even walk if you have to) for one minute then you repeat the sprint, again going all out. This will prove very challenging and at first you will probably only be able to repeat this cycle 3-4 times. Work your way up to 10 repetitions. You should continually challenge yourself to go faster. The slow period is very important as well so be sure to time it accurately. Don't push too hard and be sure you are ready (at the right level of fitness).

If your activity is an elliptical machine the same applies. Set it to the highest setting and go all out for each sprint. It is easier to do the sprints in activities such as running, cycling or swimming so I would encourage you to choose one of these. Running is probably the most beneficial for overall fitness as it improves bone density and balance. However, you should be careful about running if you have back or knee problems. The next best option, in my opinion, is to take up cycling.

If you are not in good shape...

If you are overweight and/or have not been exercising at first this activity will be difficult. I would suggest you start on an elliptical machine or a bicycle. Warm up for 10 minutes. Increase the resistance on the machine to a high setting and go as hard as you can for one minute. Bring it back down to a comfortable level that will allow you to catch your breath and use this setting for one minute or up to two minutes (but no longer) if you are very short of breath. When you can do this comfortably for 10 cycles you are ready to start running. You will lose weight and gain strength rapidly.

This may be difficult at first if you are out of shape. However, with patience and perseverance the benefits will far outweigh the initial efforts. You will be in such great shape and will begin to feel better than you have perhaps felt in years. And remember, anything worth doing requires discipline. So please stay with it, in the end you'll be happy you did!

Now back to the exercise. As you work on your endurance pay close attention to your body. If you are in any pain other than muscle soreness slow down the pace. You can change activity either for variety or to find which one you like best. You should feel worked but you should not feel sick or be unable to do your normal daily activities.

As you become accustomed to the work you will develop your own rhythm. The key to improvement is to push yourself. You are investing the time so you should use it effectively. Doing your endurance sessions with the sprints (this is often referred to as High Intensity Interval Training or HIIT) will increase your fitness to levels you may never have known you could reach. This in turn will add years of health to your life.

Strength

In the old days man became strong in the course of daily life. Strength was required to live. Today our lifestyle affords very little opportunity to become strong unless you work at a job that demands physical strength. If you are ill it is very likely that you are weak and not paying much attention to strength.

Many people have very little strength, especially as they age. Strength is essential as it is the foundation for holding our bodies together. Core strength creates the tone that holds our body together at rest and during any kind of movement. Strength creates denser bones and ligaments that are capable of withstanding daily body stress with minimal effort.

There are many other benefits. It helps maintain proper levels of hormones such as testosterone and improves metabolic rate. It produces endorphins which themselves contribute to a series of benefits. I contend that with all we know we have only touched the tip of the iceberg in understanding the benefits of building strength.

That it is beneficial has been largely recognized and along with the recognition many ways to develop strength have been developed. There are a multitude of methods with different objectives (body building, athletic performance, recovery/rehabilitation, general fitness). If you are already into fitness you have probably ventured into some of these methods. Depending on your objectives you should reevaluate your methods.

Here we'll discuss building strength as you recover from illness as well as building and maintaining strength for life. The methods are geared towards building a balanced core for overall fitness. Specialty movements such as those used for body building are great for building muscle mass but are poor contributors to overall fitness and efficient body function. If your goal is recovery and excellent fitness (and good athletic performance) the strength program will do wonders for you.

The program will work well for everyone from beginner to the most advanced. As you progress there are various methods of increasing the effort and thus strength. The beauty of this program is that you can perform it almost anywhere. No weights are required (there is one small exception). It is easy to fit into any schedule. This is a key component to making it work.

There are many reasons why this program is as it is. The most important is that it has been thoroughly tested and has proven to be an effective strength building programs. If you are the curious type feel free to experiment but be careful and take time to learn. If you stick with it you'll benefit substantially. You will feel it and you will see it. Quite appealing is that it consumes only about 2 hours each week.

If you want to measure progress re-assess yourself at least once every 6 months to see how well you are doing. Of course the mirror and your overall enhanced feeling of wellbeing will be your best indicators of progress.

The Program

The program consists of a basic set of exercises performed in three different workout formats. Each format has its specific purpose and goals. The key is that the basic movements are the same and this will allow you to learn their proper form and remember them with little effort. Here are the exercises in their execution sequence:

1. Core circuit:

    a. Cyclist's bends

    b. Abdominal crunches

    c. Side twists

2. Simple squat

3. Single leg heel raises

4. Kettle bell swings (core)

5. Wide hand pushups (palms facing away)

6. Wide grip pull ups (palms facing away)

7. Lateral raises (with weights or exercise bands)

8. Iso-tension arm curl/extension

That's it. The sequence should be performed twice weekly with two rest days in between (for example: Monday and Thursday, Tuesday and Friday, Wednesday and Saturday). Each session you should alternate with one of the three workout formats. The exercises are described in Appendix C.

I have been doing this sequence for years. It is always tough and always causes some degree of muscle soreness as an indicator of its effectiveness. Every person that tries it has good things to say about it and best of all the results are phenomenal and almost instant.

The three workout formats add variation to reduce boredom but more importantly they keep the muscles 'confused' which improves their effectiveness. They are based on solid principles that have proven to be some of the most effective forms of exercising. Following is a brief description of each format.

Base Repetition

This is the form of exercise most commonly used and known to all of us. It consists of executing one exercise movement repeatedly for a number of repetitions against enough resistance to cause muscle failure when the repetitions are completed. At this point a short period of rest is undertaken and then the exercise is repeated again in sets of repetitions for a predetermined number of sets.

This format is the oldest form of resistance and strength building exercise. If you have ever been to a gym you'll notice that this is what most people are doing.

The benefit of this format is that you focus on one movement at a time and you can easily adjust the resistance load to your level. Even though you are exerting yourself until failure (or near failure) you have time to recover between sets.

In movements where we are not using weights the manner of increasing the load for each movement is based on speed of execution and rest between sets. I will elaborate more below.

Circuit sets

This form of exercise consists of executing the exercises in groups one after the other without rest until one set of each exercise has been performed. This is one circuit. Each circuit is followed by a short rest and then repeated.

Circuit training creates strength endurance. It taxes your cardiovascular system while also building strength. You will breathe harder and sweat more when you do circuits.

Super slow

This is the toughest form of executing the exercises and requires additional mental focus. It is my personal favorite form of exercise as it builds strength coupled with an added dose of mental discipline. It requires executing each movement very slowly. Doing so requires focus and strength and reduces the possibility of injury while requiring you to use very strict form.

Each exercise is executed using very slow repetitions that last at least 6 to 10 seconds during each phase of the exercise. Thus, when doing a push up for example, it takes 6-10 seconds to go down immediately followed by 6-10 seconds to return to the starting point. 8 to10 repetitions are performed in this manner without pause. Believe me, this is tough! At first it is likely that you will have to do a simplified form of each exercise (explained later) until you build up the strength required to do these. When done properly you will do only one set of each exercise during this workout and never more than two.

By using these three forms of doing a simple set of exercises you continually keep the body 'on it's toes' while becoming adept at executing each exercise using perfect form. This maximizes progress while reducing the possibility of injury.

Rest

Without rest we would not be able to function. It is the most important aspect of healing and recovery. It regulates mood and mental awareness. It allows the body to rebuild itself. The body is designed to spend at least 1/3 of its life resting, a sure indicator of the importance of rest. Not getting enough rest will make you sick.

Likewise, getting too much rest is also bad. Too much rest and your body will begin to lose tissue and bone density. You will gain weight and develop lethargy. Brain function is impaired. You become frail and vulnerable to the environment. In short, too much is just as bad as too little. The majority of people, however, do not get enough rest. Modern day life tends to keep people going well beyond their limits. And this stress will hurt you.

The body operates in accordance with a natural rhythm/cycle. At the start of the day it is in 'purge' mode, riding itself of waste. Fluid consumption is particularly important at this point (that is why you drink immediately upon rising).

During the middle of the day it is in 'operation' mode, exhibiting energy and alertness. Within this cycle it is often a good thing to take a short nap (usually early afternoon around 3PM). Most people feel the need to nap naturally around this time.

In the evening you enter 'recovery' mode. This is incudes evening wind down and sleep. You should allow your body this time to recover and reenergize itself for the following day.

We have a tendency to ignore the cycles and force our way through the day. Energy drinks are quite popular to provide a boost. None of these things are good if they are done on a regular basis. If you are ill and recovering these are definitely not allowed.

To heal you must sleep well and regularly. Rest whenever your body is asking you for rest. Make rest something you look forward to. Here are some suggestions for a restful sleep:

- Keep it regular
  Sleep and wake at the same time everyday. Avoid sleeping in. My father sleeps with the day, awakening at dawn's light and going to bed at dusk. He is 85 and extremely healthy. While this is ideal (it aligns perfectly with our natural rhythm) it is not required. A regular schedule is.

- Take a warm bath
  A warm bath with Epsom salts and essential oils is soothing to the body and the mind.

    o Do not be rushed.

- o   Use water at around 90 degrees.

- o   Bathe right before bed. It is great to get under the covers after a warm bath.

- o   Allow your mind to relax by focusing on breathing.

- o   Practice visualization or meditate while bathing.

- Keep the bedroom cool and dark
  The ideal room temperature for sleeping is quite cool. Generally it is somewhere between 60-68 degrees. I personally set the thermostat to 72 and I have a ceiling fan circulating the air in my bedroom. Keep the room as dark as possible as even small amounts of light can disturb the body's sleep cycle.

- Use quality linen
  Buy organic linen from one of the sources listed in Appendix C. As stated in the next chapter most linen has toxins and is also not comfortable. You have these against your skin for 8 hours everyday. They should be the best that you can afford. Use a high thread count, natural fiber without any additives, coatings or colors.

- Take melatonin
  If you are over 50 you should definitely take melatonin, especially if you have difficulty sleeping or are a light sleeper. Melatonin is produced naturally during the sleep cycle. Production diminishes as you get older.

Your daily activities also influence your sleep. Fresh air, sunshine and exercise are particularly beneficial.

Once you start doing this you will be amazed at how it changes you. Note that you should ALWAYS exercise with caution. Take your time and DO NOT push yourself. There should be a level of exertion but you should increase it slowly as you acquire strength and your body becomes accustomed to the exercise. You will know this by the level of soreness. Mild muscle soreness is OK and normal but it should never interfere with your activities.

If you are ill, use judgment to determine how to proceed. Move slowly at first until your body starts getting stronger. It's OK if at first all you can do is just breathe. Start there. As you progress you will know when you are ready to do more. Listen to your body.

Problems/Joint Pain

Joint problems, particularly knee related, are common. Generally, they are an indication that surrounding muscle is too weak, that we have suffered an injury, or that we have a bad physical habit that is stressing the joint. When left unattended these lead to chronic problems that, in today's world, results in surgery.

If you suffer from joint issues here is my suggested course of action.

1. If there is no swelling, apply a heated caster oil pack to the ailing joint daily until it improves.

2. If the joint is swollen, ice it down to reduce the swelling and move it gently while it is numbed from the icing.

3. Start exercising the surrounding muscles. It is a good idea to speak with a physical therapist to understand how to do this, as there are many possibilities.

4. Work slowly. If the pain is the result of tendonitis your best remedy is to allow the joint to rest. Move it without resistance during this time.

Muscular aches and soreness subside on their own as you become accustomed to exercise. Massage is helpful to speed up recovery and wellness.

6 Cleaning Your Space

"Your greatest exposure to toxic substances is right in your own home. Sometimes it's hardest to see what is closest to you, what you see every day."

Debra Lynn Dadd

Your home should be your haven, a place of peace and comfort. It should be safe, cozy and conducive to your wellbeing both mentally and physically. Yet today's homes are far from that. Yes, they often look beautiful, tidy and inviting. But that comfy looking couch is oozing formaldehyde and flame-retardants, at least. That carpet you walk on bare-footed is letting off benzene, acetone and a bunch of other toxins. And we haven't even looked at your soap (not really soap, notice they're called things like 'bath bars', 'body wash', etc.), shampoo, toothpaste, cleaners, etc.

Toxicity is killing many more people than can be counted. Since it is hiding all around you in such innocent looking items you don't even notice what's happening. Things were bad in the early 90s when I started looking into this. Today they are much worse, along with increased incidents of cancers, autoimmune disorders and ailments that go by unnoticed until they become something major.

Take notice. Here in the US the policy for using chemicals and man-made materials is one of 'Good until proven bad'. This means that products are produced and delivered to consumers with minimal proof of their long-term effects. By the time the damage is done many people have suffered. Never assume safety with new products. ALWAYS look for products that are produced with natural materials.

If you want to be healthy you will more than likely have to turn your home inside out. I will guide you through some basics here but urge you to look up the references and take action to make your home your safe haven.

Personal Care

Each day you use a variety of items to take care of personal hygiene. If you are like most modern day Americans your bathroom is loaded with all sorts of wonderful smelling, smooth feeling things that you just love... And they are hurting you.

The commercial focus on personal items is based on how they look, feel and smell, not how they affect you. You would be sold motor oil as a moisturizer if it smelled good. Very little attention is paid to providing you products that are actually good for you.

Of course the marketing team is there to convince you otherwise. In the end no one really cares about your wellbeing as long as they get your money. This is what capitalism and the 'wealth' mindset does.

To be fair there are good products made by good people. But these people don't have the marketing muscle or the production power of the big guys so, unless you are looking, you are likely to pass their products by.

As we become more aware of the implications of these products on our health things are changing. It is still tricky and confusing. Many businesses are using the health-oriented buzzwords while still providing garbage. Just because it is sold at the health food store doesn't mean it's healthy.

Soap/Shampoo

Most of us bathe daily, using some form of 'soap' and shampoo to do so. For thousands of years bathing consisted only of water. Somewhere along the way it was discovered that we could make water wetter by using saponified[28] fats.

Modern day commercial soaps are no longer really soap. They are more like detergents with added chemicals to give off their smooth texture and aroma. As a matter of fact, they cannot legally be called soap[29]. Glycerin, a primary ingredient of real soap is removed and used in many other ways that produce more income. It is replaced with chemicals that lather synthetically and can be sold to you for less. You are bathing in chemicals that are absorbed by your skin and are likely causing problems that you aren't even aware are related to this stuff you're using.

It's a catch-22. Using these glycerin-depleted detergents dries your skin so you wind up buying moisturizers and lotions from companies who have purchased the glycerin that was originally in the soap. They've repackaged it into yet another product and are now selling it back to you.

---

[28] Soap is made by combining a fat with an alkali.
[29] The term 'soap' is regulated and cannot be used unless it is real soap. Good luck finding any soap in a supermarket.

Real soap is amazing. It is made with real oils and salt (alkali). It is healthy for you and beneficial. Yet most of the people I've worked with have never actually used real soap. It is important to use real soap for various reasons:

- Ingredients are pure and natural

- It nurtures the skin and the body

- It is a carrier of essential oils

- It smells and feels wonderful without the use of chemicals

- It eliminates the need for moisturizers and skin lotions

You can purchase real soap in bar form and in liquid form. I personally prefer Dr. Bronner's (liquid castile soap) as it is pure and has a multitude of uses. I use it as a bathing soap, shampoo and shaving cream. It can even be used as toothpaste!

You can choose other soaps as long as they are 100% Pure. For the most part the best real soap is locally made. You can find it in health food stores and at farmer's markets. It is more expensive than the supermarket detergents you are probably used to, but its your only choice to stay healthy.

Hair conditioner/after shave lotion

Just as there is almost no real soap available commercially, the same holds true for hair conditioners. They suffer from the same issues as those detergent products used for bathing.

The same is true of after-shave lotions. Skin is also more sensitive and absorbent after shaving so that makes things worse.

My product of choice here is organic apple cider vinegar. It is a great product. It has many uses; among them it can be used as both hair conditioner and as an after-shave lotion. To use it mix it with filtered water at a 50/50 ratio.

As a conditioner, mix it into your hair liberally, allow it to sit for a minute or two, and then rinse. Contrary to what you may think, it leaves no odor once it is dry.

As an after-shave lotion apply it to your skin after shaving. It will sting just as any after-shave lotion would; only it is great for your skin. Ideally, let it dry. Or you can rinse it after you've applied it for a few seconds. It does wonders for your skin.

Modern toothpaste is also toxic. Fluoride, aspartame, DEA, propylene glycol, ... the list goes on. These toxins enter your bloodstream through your mouth, one of the most absorbent areas of your body. The typical American does this every day, multiple times per day, for most of their lives. Then, as if this weren't enough, many also add a chemical mouthwash!

On top of that most modern day tooth problems are related to diet. If you eat well your teeth will not decay, you will not have gum issues and your smile will last you a lifetime.

Brushing your teeth and keeping them healthy is simple. Brush with a dab of baking soda. Rinse and then apply 3-6 drops of food grade peroxide to the brush and brush again. Do not rinse. This will do wonders for your teeth and mouth. You will never use toothpaste again (nor will you ever have another cavity). If you would like a more elaborate recipe Appendix A has recipes for full, pasty toothpaste like most are accustomed to.

There may be some all-natural commercial toothpaste that is healthy. I haven't tried any. If you venture out for something that is commercially available be sure to do your research. If you are ill do not buy anything and use the basic brushing with baking soda and food grade peroxide.

Then there are deodorants. First of all, the fact that we find something as natural as sweat undesirable is sad. Even though excessive sweating (or lack of sweating) may be a symptom of a problem, generally sweat is produced to regulate body temperature in response to our environment.

Odor is caused when sweat comes in contact with skin bacteria. Excessive skin bacteria (from lack of bathing, for example) are often the cause of odor, not necessarily sweat itself.

So to minimize odor from sweating minimize skin bacteria. One way to accomplish that naturally is to use mineral salts. Use baking soda as an underarm skin powder to reduce perspiration and bacteria. Mineral salts can be applied with a mineral salt deodorant block.

Other items like nail polish or hair color should be avoided. If you must, use them only if you are not ill, and then do so sparingly. While you are healing you will not be coloring your hair or using nail polish or any other product other than those listed above. No exceptions.

Household

Most households today are loaded with man-made toxins. Couches, mattresses, cleaners, etc. are all killers. Do a little online research and you will see the poisons lurking in your home. The same holds true for most household cleaners.

One of the best things you can do is ventilate your home. Allowing as much fresh air to circulate through your home removes toxins that are in the air, such as formaldehyde and other solvents.

As an alternative, if you cannot ventilate your home regularly (such as when you live up north in winter), indoor plants absorb many toxins and freshen air. They beautify your home and for many are a great hobby[30].

As for actually removing toxins from your home, there are many choices you can make as to the materials used for household items. The details around this are beyond the scope of what we're covering here (refer to the references in Appendix C) but here are a few things to consider.

Household carpeting is extremely toxic. Even carpets made with natural fibers become the home of dust mites and bacteria. If possible get rid of all carpeting and replace it with natural wood floors or tiles. If you must live in a home with carpets DO NOT walk barefoot.

Furnishings made of particleboard are much cheaper than real wood furnishings but give off fumes and toxins from the adhesives and chemicals used during construction. This is a major source of air toxicity. Choose real wood with natural adhesives.

Be wary of anything that touches your skin. Using starch on your clothing or 'iron-free' fabrics is exposing yourself to harsh chemicals that can be causing harm you aren't even aware of.

You must rid yourself of all cleaners that are not made 100% from the following ingredients:

- o   castile soap

- o   borax

---

[30] There is substantial evidence that shows the therapeutic benefits of gardening and working with plants.

- o distilled vinegar

- o baking soda

- o hydrogen peroxide

- o essential oils

- o citrus

It is quite easy to use the above to make any household cleaner. I encourage you to do so. IF you cannot use a 100% organic product do not use any at all. This is important! Appendix C has a few of my favorite remedies that you should start using immediately. If you research some of the websites in Appendix D you will find many other excellent remedies that will contribute to your health and wellbeing while keeping your home clean and safe.

Do not use commercial pesticides. Instead use natural pesticides that you can purchase or make yourself. Some great ingredients are:

- o Garlic

- o Chile pepper (powder)

- o Diatomaceous earth

- o Borax

- o Baking soda

- o Citrus oil

Use these ingredients to create pesticides that will do the job and keep you and your loved ones safe. Appendix C has a few recipes to get you started.

Your House, Your Home

This short chapter outlines some of the most critical aspects of making your home a healthy and safe place to be. Your home should be a refuge that nurtures and fortifies you, a place of rest and comfort. Yet in today's modern world it seems that homes are more of a status symbol than a place of comfort. We've given up essentials and substituted them with useless symbols that are poor at best, harmful at most.

I hope these words have inspired, enlightened and given you the things you need to truly provide meaning to 'Home Sweet Home'. On the path to healing and health it is important to have a place where everything leads to harmony. I know this sounds very 'cliché' but there is truth to it and I certainly hope you'll see that.

7   Your Mind and Healing

"The intuitive mind is a sacred gift and the rational mind is a faithful servant. We have created a society that honors the servant and has forgotten the gift."
Albert Einstein

For many years humanity has considered its ability to think to be the grand characteristic that sets us humans apart from all other living creatures on this planet. We attribute our 'advanced' state of being to self-consciousness and our ability to rationalize and deduce. While this does distinguish us from other living creatures I argue that it has not necessarily made us any better. On the contrary, many of our problems and the manner in which we have become a 'plague' to our own planet show that our ability to think is killing us.

Our mind's constant bantering over everything that makes up our life is constantly causing us to make choices out of incorrect assumptions and rationale. Over the history of humanity there are endless examples of how thinking has led to 'wrong' actions, massive destruction and immense suffering. Today things are no different. Take one look at every crisis that plagues us; you will see that they are all the result of 'thinking' and rationalizing.

Our 'mind' can be a great asset as the ability to think and rationalize to resolve some predicaments is a good thing. The problem comes from allowing our mind to become 'us'. Descartes made a grand mistake when he stated, 'I think, therefore I am'[31]. Today we continue to propagate that mistake, resulting in a slow and complete destruction of our world and, if it isn't stopped, our race. Of course our world will recover. It was here long before us and will return to balance after we are gone.

The largest drawback of our thinking mind is that it shifts us from 'experiencing' to reflecting upon what we 'think', via cognition, an experience is. This is not the same and produces a very different result in our physical world, affecting our body and the things around us. For example, reading about the dangers of sharks in the ocean causes many

---

[31] Quieting the mind through meditation clearly shows that we can stop thinking and still be. We are not our thoughts.

of us to have a fear of going for a swim and enjoying the wonderful physical (and relaxing) sensation of that experience when, in reality, it is rare to be attacked by a shark and, for those of us who have had the experience, denies us the experience of observing and enjoying the beauty of these magnificent creatures, not to mention the pleasant experience of swimming in the ocean.

Our mind is the main cause for many of our fears. Worrying, obsessions, negative thoughts, unrealistic expectations are all inventions of our minds and obstacles to experiencing and living in the real world. Eventually these things manifest themselves physically in everything from high blood pressure to cancer to mental disorders (obsessive compulsion, depression, anxiety, etc.) causing further mental disturbance and further deterioration.

Our current obsession with possessions and wealth are good examples of the destructive effects of thinking. Society has programmed our minds to think that these have to be major goals in

> "If you weren't happy yesterday, you won't be happy tomorrow. Money is not happiness."
>
> Mark Cuban

our lives. The 'American Dream' is nothing more than a false mental fantasy. It has nothing to do with happiness and joy. But our minds are constantly telling us (thanks to mass media advertising and Hollywood) that this must be a primary goal in order for us to achieve joy. The number of unhappy people that live in a big house and drive BMWs along with the number of unhappy people (sacrificing their lives) trying to own a big house and drive BMWs probably accounts for over 80% of the population. And all of this because our thinking minds have completely taken over us, blinding us to our true desires and the simple things that would make our lives so much more rewarding.

Remember that, as physical beings, our ultimate goal is to 'feel' good and be sensory fulfilled. Achieving this fulfillment would bring us joy and enable us to go through life happily. Our mind can help this cause or inhibit it. In today's world it mostly serves to inhibit rather than help and facilitate. To achieve joy and fulfillment as human beings we have to change that.

This need to shut down mental dominance is so true that many people recur to drugs, alcohol, mindless sex (pornography) and other escapes from the mind to find peace and a (temporary) sense of pleasure. Of course, being that this is a temporary fix, the mind eventually returns, inflicting its grieving program on us. This is the root cause of addiction and all of its related problems (crime and suicide).

Joy, happiness, and our fulfillment as human beings can be achieved by quieting the mind. While it is difficult to do for those that have never experienced it, imagine that you could just stop thinking. Yep, just imagine that you can turn off the mind and no thought, nothing, passed through your mind. Even though this experience may seem inconceivable to you it is perfectly possible and practiced by a growing number of people every day.

Now imagine that when you do think, the thoughts that fill your mind are only the thoughts that you want there. No worrying thoughts, no negativity, nothing that would make you feel bad or afraid. Again, this is perfectly possible and practiced by many every day. Doing this makes your mind your servant and not the other way around as it more than likely is at this moment. This here is the key to life and happiness. It is the enlightenment that the Buddha found, and can be arguably viewed as the true ultimate life goal.

If there is only one thing you get out of this book it should be this: learn to quiet the mind. The clarity of sense and direction that you will achieve, the discipline that you will be able to command, the peace that you will obtain, the discipline and focus that you will have, the complete detachment from all things material... you will be free in a way that I cannot explain.

Shortly, I will tell you exactly what you need to do to get there. Your job will be to follow through and persist until you do. Once you get a taste of quieting your mind your life will change forever. There is absolutely nothing else like this.

However quieting the mind is not an easy thing to learn how to do. Once you learn it telling your mind to shut up on demand will be easy. But getting there will be tough. Your mind will fight you every step of the way. Detaching yourself from your thoughts is not something your consciousness (or modern day society and its slew of organized dictators, themselves lost to their mental faculties) wants you to do. So there is a large chance that you will never get to this place. I urge you to work at it regardless of how long it may take. There is nothing more rewarding.

As a child you once had this ability. But it was slowly taken away from you. Our education system, the media, those around you (they don't know any better) all worked consistently to build the thoughts that govern you, by telling you what was good or bad, right or wrong. By limiting your creativity and fitting you into a life filled with rules of do's and don'ts. Now it is time to undo all of that. So let us begin.

We will reach our goal by starting with familiar activities, some of which we are already practicing (you are doing that morning session we introduced in 'Immediate Actions' and working on your breathing aren't you?). The process we are going to follow consists of three steps:

- Concentration
  We will first learn to concentrate. The average person has an attention span of less than 10 seconds. This is bad. It is the primary cause why people are so easily distracted and sidetracked. It causes accidents, inability to learn, anxiety and a host of other problems. When you implement my suggestions you will get to the point where you can concentrate for hours.

- Meditation
  Once you learn to concentrate we will use that capability to quiet the mind. This is true meditation. The term meditation is somewhat of a misnomer as it implies pondering upon something whereas true meditation as we shall learn is to completely quiet the conscious mind (i.e. to stop thinking). We will begin our exploration of meditation in this section and will discuss it further in chapter 8.

- Visualization
  When coupled with focused, deliberate thought, concentration opens the doors to changing our beliefs and ridding ourselves of thoughts (conscious and unconscious) that contribute to negativity. This is the core of joy and key to the discovery and achievement of our true desires.

I can't stress enough the importance of persistence as you develop your mental skills. At first it will be difficult and frustrating, as your mind does not want to be tamed! It is amazing the games that go on within our heads and this process will bring them out in full force. So before we get to the exercises themselves here are a few things to keep in mind:

- Observe your thoughts as you learn to concentrate. As you go through your day and you notice yourself wandering from your objective return to what you are doing. You will find yourself wandering less and less.

- Some of the thoughts you hear yourself echoing in your head will seem very real. You will perceive the need to scratch, move, drink, sneeze, and everything imaginable. To make sure these aren't real be sure to drink, use the restroom and sit comfortably before you start.

- Find a location that has no distraction. Turn off your phone, music and any other source of distraction.

- Habit is good. Try to use the same location, time and conditions. This will make it easier as we are all creatures of habit.

- When you are done with the exercise spend a few minutes pondering what just happened. At this point it is OK to think!

Did I mention persistence? Oh I did. Then let the journey begin.

Concentration

To concentrate is to keep one's full attention focused on one thing and only one thing to the exclusion of all others. Many of us have experienced moments of acute focus, usually at a trying moment, throughout our lives. These moments are often associated with an instance in our lives where we were required to perform an action that had a lot of meaning. For example, the person who somehow manages to maneuver their car out of a seemingly inescapable accident will attest to a moment in which the world seems to stand still. The athlete in the midst of making a great play will attest to a similar moment. This is concentration. Perhaps a more familiar moment is the moment of sexual orgasm. During that instant the entire world seems to cede completely to the intensity of what is occurring.

While we will often claim to be "concentrating" on something the truth is the average person can only hold their focus for about 5-10 seconds. Try it to see how well you fare. Do the following exercise:

Using a watch or clock with a second hand focus your attention on the second hand as it moves. Think only of the second hand and watch as it moves. Within moments of starting to do this you will see how your mind starts interjecting other thoughts. How many seconds passed before the first thought led you off? You may still be looking at the second hand moving but your thought is no longer there.

We will make this our first exercise. It is good to have a watch with a second hand, as this will allow you to practice often. Persistence will pay off.

Learning to concentrate
Sit comfortably wherever you are (at home, on a work break, in a taxi, on the bus or train, in a plane – all of these are good locations to practice). Take a few slow deep breaths as you learned in part one. Bring your attention to the watch and, more specifically, to the second hand. Just follow it. Do not count or ponder any thought. The only thing on your mind at this moment is the second hand.

Within a short period (seconds at first) your mind will begin to wander. As soon as you notice this happening just bring your focus back to the second hand. Continue doing this for 5 minutes. Eventually you will be able to do it for the entire 5 minutes without losing focus. At this point you are beginning to learn what it means to concentrate.

You should do this exercise at least twice each day without failure. The more you do it the sooner you will begin to focus and learn what it is to concentrate. You will also notice this in your other activities. It is good to learn to focus on whatever you're doing. For example, when driving focus solely on driving rather than going through your to do list or what you'll be having for dinner. When eating focus on eating, etc. This will all seem counter intuitive at first as you are used to using your mental time differently. But as you get used to it you'll notice a reduction in stress, anxiety and a clearer sense of thinking. You'll start to see little things like an improved ability to solve problems.

If you've ever been to a Buddhist temple or retreat you will notice that the monks practice simple tasks and do so in silence. They are focusing the mind on the task at hand and freeing themselves of other conscious thoughts. This is a common practice to them as they seek to spend as much time as possible in the 'white space' between thoughts, a concept that is foreign to many of us. Learning to concentrate will give you an understanding of this and as you move forward (persistence) you will come to see the wonder and power of this. Right now I can only ask you to bear with me and follow through.

Back to the exercise; you should continue doing this until you can focus without once being distracted from watching the second hand. This will take you anywhere from 3 to 6 months depending on how diligent and disciplined you are. Yes, this seems like a long time but remember your mind has been playing games with you for a long time and it will take you some time to show it who's boss. The benefits are immediate and cumulative as you progress so you will notice improvements in many areas of thought.

Focused breathing

Now that you are in charge of your mind (at least for a short period) you can start expanding on your dominance. This exercise is essentially the same as the first except that you will now focus solely on your breath. Watch yourself inhale and exhale and, just as before, if your mind wanders bring it back to your breath. Close your eyes, as this will help your focus.

You should start doing this at least twice a day whenever you have any idle time and can sit quietly. Do it for as long as you can. For example, for the duration of your taxi or bus ride to work. It is a good idea to have a timer or some other form of breaking the focus since you will tend to lose track of time (which is precisely our objective and a good indicator of progress). If you are doing it mornings and evenings (a common practice) go for a minimum of 10 minutes knowing that more is better.

You should continue with this practice for another 6 months. At the end of this time you should be able to focus solely on your breath at will for periods of up to 30 minutes. This becomes a very enjoyable task and something you will look forward to, again a good sign that you are progressing in the right direction. At this point many of your friends and acquaintances should have noticed a difference in your demeanor and general composure.

As you can see learning to concentrate is a simple task that requires much discipline to dominate. It is no wonder many never even come close to doing so regardless of the benefits that can be outlined. It is sad that most people are not disciplined enough to do this. So again, be persistent. The reward far outweighs the initial effort.

A note on the practice of Yoga

I want to take a moment to talk about yoga. No doubt that you have heard, seen and perhaps even tried it once or twice. Or perhaps you have made it a part of your daily practice. In speaking with many practitioners and even certified yoga teachers I often see that many are missing the point. So I'd like to speak on the objectives of yoga and offer some guidelines for its practice.

Many people believe that yoga is a form of physical exercise. While this is true to some extent the physical aspects of yoga are a vehicle towards the discipline of quieting the mind. The ultimate goal of yoga is to achieve what is called enlightenment (more on this in chapter 8). Enlightenment is achieved via the quieting of the mind, the freeing of thoughts. This is yoga's ultimate purpose.

Unknown to many there are methods of yoga that do not even require physical exercise. However, since for most of us the easiest thing to focus on is a physical distraction the most popular forms of yoga all include physical exercise. Focusing on a yoga pose and breathing give the mind something to 'do' as it is disciplined. The intensity of a pose requires concentration for its proper execution. In the process the mind frees itself of unwanted thoughts as we learn to 'let go' and settle into each pose.

If we practice yoga and keep this focus its full benefits will be achieved. Otherwise it largely becomes a form of stretching and conditioning, not bad things but short of the ultimate goal. If you are investing the time it is my hope that you will invest it fully.

Meditation

After you have achieved dominance of your thoughts the next step is to completely quiet the mind, or meditate. It is important that you have followed the preceding guidance and have achieved the ability to focus your mind, as this is critical to achieving the state of meditation. This means that, on average, you have been practicing the concentration exercises for 6 months to a year.

You may, of course, attempt to quiet the mind at any point once you understand the goal and the concept of not thinking. Without the ability to concentrate you will more than likely become frustrated. Therefore it is better to attempt this when you are ready. Only you can really have an idea of when you are ready so feel free to try as often as you wish. If you are not successful please continue with the concentration exercises. I believe I have mentioned that persistence is key!

Different things happen when you stop thinking, the most notable being the loss of the concept of time. Whether you meditate for 5 minutes or 2 hours you won't feel the difference. Once the mind is quiet it is as if time stops.

A second event that I experience is what I call the observation of thought. You will see the things that are going through your unconscious mind as if you were watching some kind of movie. You will see 'thoughts' you didn't know you had passing before you at a very fast rate. When this happens it is important to not follow any of these thoughts as that is a return to thinking. This will happen though, and when it does you should return to being quiet immediately.

You may have other experiences. Some people describe seeing a kaleidoscope of color and others see amorphous forms. It is important to make sure that this is not thought. You will know.

Quieting the Mind

At first you should find a location that is peaceful where you will not be distracted or interrupted. Eventually you will be able to do this almost anywhere but at first it will be much easier if you avoid any potential inhibitors.

Start by sitting (or lying) comfortably. I sit on a yoga cushion called a 'zafu'[32] and use a relaxed lotus position. If you are at work or on the bus then just sit straight and place your feet flat on the ground. At busy locations I have even escaped to the restroom and meditated in a stall. Once you learn how to quiet the mind you will be able to do it almost anywhere. I usually meditate for a few minutes before important meetings or presentations.

Once you are comfortable turn your attention to your breath as you learned to do in the concentration exercises. Relax your entire body as your breathing becomes slower and deeper.

As you reach the meditative state you will naturally lose your thought (of breathing). The first few times you do this you may not be able to become completely quiet. Keep working at it. When thought vanishes you will know. Time will seem to stop.

Your first experience of this moment is likely to take you out of it. Most people will experience this 'aha' moment in a euphoric way and will get excited over what has just occurred, losing the moment. This is OK. It is a wonderful feeling to finally get here. When this happens just go back and find it again. You will begin to find this place and stay here for ever-longer periods. It will take some time to get into the groove of meditating but each experience will leave you yearning for the next one. After a few months of this you should be able to stay in a meditative state for periods of 20 to 30 minutes without once ever returning to thought.

---

[32] Appendix C provides purchasing references.

As you will lose your concept of time I strongly suggest that you use a timer. My watch has a timer (these days you are more likely to use a smartphone timer) and I usually set it prior to starting. When you have the time it is good to allow yourself to go until you naturally 'come back' to your thoughts. It is good to keep track of how long these periods last. Over time they should get longer. When I first started these periods would naturally last between 20-30 minutes. Today they can go on for over three hours.

The effects of meditation are many. After each session you should observe how you feel and enjoy the 'lightness' that follows. This renewed feeling is something that you will never grow tired of.

It will easily take you one to two years to get to this state of quietness or 'bliss'. Be persistent. This will transform you.

Visualization

Learning to concentrate and quiet the mind is transformational for many reasons. Some of the most obvious of these are the ability to eliminate worrying and negative thoughts. But these are generally passive effects. It is possible to actively use this skill to direct productive thoughts into our mind and to change fundamental processes by 'embedding' thought patterns into our subconscious mind[33].

There are many studies and research that clearly show how our subconscious thoughts orchestrate our lives. There are also many techniques and therapy methods geared at uncovering subconscious thoughts and changing them as a form of correcting destructive and unproductive behavioral patterns. While most of these are effective they can all be greatly enhanced by the ability to quiet the mind. This is one reason why this skill is so important. Many years of therapy can be easily eliminated when we are able to focus our thoughts or shut them up at will.

Let us explore this for clarity. Sit down comfortably in a quiet place where you won't be interrupted. Now go back to a moment in your life that was extremely unpleasant. This could be a fight or a moment when you became very angry or scared. As you recall this experience focus on remembering every detail of it. Who was there, what was said and done. Essentially relive it in your mind.

---

[33] This is similar to how hypnosis works. I have not worked with hypnosis for illness but it may be helpful.

Notice how this is affecting you. You heart rate is elevated and your breathing is faster. You are essentially bringing that moment back into your body just by reliving it in your mind.

Now lets change the thought. Think of a moment in which you were extremely happy and full of joy. A moment in which life was perfect and you felt safe and secure. Again, relive the moment in your bind. Remember everything you can about it and how it made you feel. After doing this for a few minutes you will again notice that all of those sensations are returning to your body. Yet the moment only exists in your mind.

Essentially what I'm saying is that your body believes everything your mind tells it. It doesn't matter whether it is real or not. If it is happening in your mind it is happening in your body. This is why worrying leads to anxiety and panic attacks. It is also often why depression happens. Thoughts trigger innumerable biochemical reactions in your body. These reactions affect your behavior.

The ability to turn thoughts off or to focus only on desirable thoughts or the activity at hand directly affects what is happening in your physical body. Think of this for a moment. Mastering the skills that you have started to work on in the previous 2 sections is the foundation for managing how you feel and how you behave.

Which leads us to visualization. By learning to visualize we set the conditions in our body for the events that we visualize. This has been done effectively for areas such as sports and addiction management for a long time. It is one of the focuses of techniques such as hypnosis and suggestive repetition.

I like to think of visualization as a form of conscious dreaming. We can tailor it to meet specific needs and elicit desired effects. It is very effective as a tool to help with healing or achieving goals.

In its simplest form visualization can be viewed as daydreaming. This is extremely healthy. Dreaming and visualizing precede action and are important to achieving goals. Ask anyone that has succeeded at something and they will all tell you that it was first a dream.

We all visualize ourselves where we'd like to be at different points throughout our lives. Our imagination is particularly vivid during childhood. As we grow up one of the things we do is temper our day dreams with what we begin to see as our reality (for example, dreaming of playing the piano may at some point become tempered by not being able to afford a piano and/or lessons or dreaming of being a famous speaker may be tempered by someone making you believe you are not smart enough).

Constructive visualization starts by envisioning every detail of what we desire. This involves using all of our senses as we visualize. As we progress we must also visualize how we are going to get there. The effect is that we begin to act as we see ourselves, progressing towards our desired goal in daily acts. But it all starts in our minds and visualizations are like a roadmap that we create as we figure out how we are going to get there.

Sweet dreams

Our first visualization exercise is one that you can use effectively every night to get a good night's sleep. Each evening as you get ready to go to bed it is helpful to rid your mind of the day's burdens. If you are a reader choose something uplifting and positive to read before bed. Mysteries and horror stories are best left to lunch or afternoon reading. The same is true if you are going to watch a movie or listen to music.

Once you are in bed and ready to close your eyes start by taking a few slow deep breaths and turning your attention to your breathing. Then, visualize yourself in a place that is pleasant and relaxing to you. This could be in a garden on a spring afternoon or by the ocean as the sun is setting. Visualize the scene with each of your senses. See it, feel it, smell it, hear it and even taste it. Be there completely. Pay no attention to time as you become more and more involved in it. This will usually take anywhere from about 5 minutes to 15 or more. Finally, within your visualization, quiet your mind. Lose all thought as you slowly drift off into your sleep. Sweet dreams!

This is one of the simplest and most effective visualizations to do. You can even go places that you've never been to; a virtual vacation! The key is to understand how by visualizing with your full attention you can command sensations so close to the real thing that you will gain almost every benefit of the actual event.

Action visualization

In this exercise our goal is to help induce a given behavior. We start by fully visualizing the desired behavior and then through small daily actions actually adapting it. We will illustrate by using dietary change as the desired outcome since for many this is a useful outcome.

Let's assume that as part of lifestyle changes you want to eat a healthier diet. Let's also assume that as part of this you want to stop eating chocolate pastries and ice cream. We also want to start eating more fruit and vegetables.

Start by finding a time and a place where you will not be interrupted or distracted. Sit comfortably in the position you normally use for your concentration/meditation. Take a few slow deep breaths and bring your focus to your breathing (notice the pattern here – we always start by telling our mind we are about to give it instruction).

Now start the visualization by first imagining yourself eating fresh fruit (choose the fruit of your liking). Savor this moment with every sense (taste, smell, see, feel, touch), all the time telling yourself how much you enjoy eating this fruit. You may eat more than one fruit if you like. At some point start seeing yourself in excellent shape, feeling strong and healthy and at your desired weight. Again, visualize this fully, all while you are enjoying your tasty fruit.

Now shift your attention to the pastries and ice cream. Visualize how they make you feel bloated, slow and sickly. Imagine yourself gaining pounds with each bite and feeling totally disgusted by this. Your stomach hurts and the smell is intolerable (imagine the worst smell possible). Again spend time here and allow your body to actually feel how terrible it feels as a result of this.

When you've had enough go back to the fruit and visualize how it instantly makes you feel better and stronger. Envision it with every sense and feel how much better your body feels as you consume this tasty fruit.

Now (in your visualization) finish eating your fruit. Sit back and enjoy how well you feel. When you are ready return your focus to your breathing and then slowly back to your real world.

As you go through your day you should always associate these same sensations with the fruit (the goodness) and also whenever you think about the pastries and ice cream (the unpleasantness).

What you are doing here is reprogramming your subconscious mind. Whatever it was you associated these items with before you are now re-associating them in a manner that is in line with your desired behavior and goals. This is the key of visualization.

Many professionals use visualization techniques to change all sorts of behaviors and do so with a high rate of success. However, in our case, since we have first learned to control our mind through concentration and meditation the power of visualization increases many times over. It is very important to first focus on concentration and meditation (in that order) as they are the true keys to change.

Use this exercise in any way desired in your life. The visualization is only limited by your imagination. Just keep in mind that the only behavior you can change is your own. Visualizing others behaving in ways that you desire does not accomplish anything! Generally speaking, you should be the only one in your visualization. You can include others so long as you are not anticipating a change in their behaviors.

This is very powerful for healing. Create a visualization that helps you find your way to better health. I will share with you the visualization I used when I was healing.

After focusing on my breath and becoming peaceful and calm I envisioned a vast ocean of crystal clear, warm water (think Caribbean). In this ocean I saw islands of sand (my tumors). I envisioned the ocean waves (healing elements) slowly breaking down these islands of sand until they were gone. I felt how these waves were so soothing and at the same time invigorating. I focused intently on their warmth and how they took the sand from the islands and made it disappear.

I did this visualization daily, multiple times, and always at bedtime. Create your visualization. Just let it come to mind and you will come up with one that works for you.

Once you get the hang of it you can use visualizations for many things and under many circumstances. Use your imagination. Your mind is a gateway to many experiences.

8 Spirituality for Healing

"The personal life deeply lived always expands into truths beyond
itself."
Anais Nin

Ask ten people what it means to be spiritual and you are likely to get ten
totally different responses. This diversity of opinions is the cause of much
controversy and even conflict today. The many leaders that intend to tell
us what it means to be spiritual further complicate things.

Regardless of the variety of views and opinions around it, being spiritual
boils down to a very fundamental set of behaviors. An exploration of the
many faces of spirituality and observation of the behaviors of the spiritual
leaders that have walked the earth allows us to create a simple definition
of spirituality that we can then use as the fundamental basis for our goals.

As we search for meaning we all wind up facing what we call spirituality.
It helps us to come to terms with things that we do not understand about
the wonders of life and the extraordinary force behind it. In essence
being spiritually connected means coming to terms with the existence of
a life force that we cannot completely define but that we know must exist
since there is no other way to explain our origin.

This 'force' is manifested in various ways. It encompasses what we call
love, enlightenment, wisdom and eternity. Turning to our spiritual leaders
we see these manifestations in the love of Jesus Christ, the
enlightenment of the Buddha and the references in all of our guiding
texts through time.

The most noticeable behavior of spirituality is that of service to others.
Without exception as we become more 'spiritual' we tend to become
more giving. We open ourselves to helping and supporting those around
us and giving more of what we have. At the same time we realize that
this brings us closer to something we cannot explain but is manifest in
the pleasant outcome of our acts. As we give, others also become more
giving, as if the effect is contagious.

A second behavior of spirituality is an inclination to care less (and often
not at all) about material possessions and outwardly influence. The
closer we get to the true force of life the more we detach ourselves from

things and impressions, learning as we go that these have no true effect on connecting us to this source of life that calls us.

As this happens a hunger develops. A hunger for understanding who we are at a deeper level. This is a turning point in our search for meaning and unknowingly turns into a quest for our better selves. This is the point at which we can say we become spiritual.

It is not possible to become spiritual just by saying so. Going to church or reading the Bible doesn't necessarily make you a spiritual being[34]. Doing these things is good and perhaps even necessary for many as a discipline and thought-provoking act. It would allow you to start pondering aspects of life and ask yourself questions, all of which are steps towards the spiritual self.

Acts of kindness, while a direct outcome of the spiritual self do not make you spiritual. Again, they will take you there as you learn to be compassionate but you must go there with your heart.

I say this because I have come across so many so called spiritual and enlightened people that believe themselves to be on some sort of spiritual realm because they practice these acts and others. It is one thing to practice these acts to fulfill an image and feed the ego, providing some kind of outward impression and self-satisfaction, and a completely different thing to truly act out of your heart with a true concern for our connectedness as human beings. Spiritual connectedness is humble, an inner journey, and it is shared through quiet acts that may go unnoticed to all but those involved. There is no ego involved in serving from the heart. And this is a big difference both to the receiver as well as the giver.

The true path to your inner self is quieting the mind. It is why we have spent such a large amount of time learning to meditate. This is the place where you connect to your greater self and, unknowingly at first, this greater self feeds you an essence that you cannot perceive. This place between thoughts is where the spirit lingers and permeates our being. This is where we commune with the greatness of life.

So how do we open the path to our spiritual selves? I've learned that the answer to this is the incorporation of simple acts into our lifestyle that eventually start to perform themselves as an inevitable outcome of spiritual awakening. However we have to be ready. If you have just

---

[34] Please do not take offense to this statement. It is sad but too often true. Self-honor and integrity matter. And it is important to look straight into our hearts and be truthful first to ourselves and then to the world around us.

started to work on the exercises in the previous chapter I strongly suggest you focus on that until you start to dominate your thoughts. In the meantime you can, of course, explore consciously via spiritual acts, reading, retreats, attending to your religious beliefs and pondering existence in the way that makes sense to you. As you progress mentally that quiet place between thoughts will begin to emerge and awakening will happen.

Meditate
I cannot stress enough the importance of daily meditation. You should continue as described in the prior chapter. If you have the time and are so inclined it is good practice to pray at the end of the session as you are calm and in a state of acceptance.

Inspirational Thought
I like to go through each day with a quote to stir up my thoughts. You can get your quotes delivered to you each day via email, or by purchasing a calendar or a book of quotes or any other means that works for you. The key here is to ponder a thought and what it means. This will develop insight into things that you may not have considered or thought of before now and will start fostering the mental outlook that leads you to your higher self.

If all of this is new to you then you may tend to think this is pointless or otherwise not worth doing. I urge you to just try it. Have each day's quote in a location where you can read it a few times a day and think about it even if you do so in passing. You will be surprised at how things work.

Over time thinking on a deeper level is something you will be more inclined to do. This is key to awakening and critical particularly for those of you that have never felt inclined to doing this. Go at your own pace and don't think of this as an obligation but rather as an act of self-discipline. It will pay off!

Acts of service
Serving is a form of achieving selflessness. Through service we develop a sense of connection with others and a sense of validity for ourselves. We make ourselves matter. This in turn triggers a whole series of slower responses towards humility and understanding.

What you do is not as important as doing it. Simple acts of chivalry (holding the door open or allowing someone into your lane while driving) are an excellent starting point. At the other end you could volunteer your weekends to being some child's 'big brother' or participating in 'Habitat for Humanity' programs.

But the simplest thing to do is to do simple things whenever you can. Help a stranger by picking up the pencil they just dropped or by allowing someone that is in a hurry to get ahead of you in the line for coffee. The key is to pay attention to what is going on around you and acting in service when you can.

Don't feel guilty if you can't. Perhaps you are late for an appointment and cannot stop to help someone jumpstart their car. As long as this is the exception and is true (you aren't convincing yourself that you are late because you really don't want to help) it is OK.

If you are ill it is likely that you have met others that are ill as well (at the doctor's office, in a hospital, church, support groups). Reach out to others in any way that you can. Something as simple as an encouraging smile does wonders.

Likewise accept help from others. Sometimes it is hard to allow yourself to receive from others. I know that is the case with me. Learning to accept the goodness of others opens your heart in another way. Allow it to happen and be thankful.

The Journey Home

"People tend to burden themselves with so many choices. But, in the
end, you can throw it all away and just make one basic, underlying
decision: Do you want to be happy, or do you not want to be happy?
It's really that simple. Once you make that choice, your path through
life becomes totally clear."

Michael A. Singer

Life is a journey, an opportunity for the soul to manifest itself physically.
When we are placed on this Earth we are given the freedom to choose,
not our circumstances, but how we respond to those circumstances.
Everything we need to make each choice we make lies before us. Our
responsibility is to choose and to choose wisely.

We can make each moment part of a joyful experience even in the face
of adversity.
What matters
is how we
respond to
that moment,
our attitude,

"Everything can be taken from a man but one thing: the last of
human freedoms - to choose one's attitude in any given set of
circumstances, to choose one's own way."

Viktor E. Frankl

nothing else. Responding compassionately and with openness is tapping
into the higher forces of life, and that energy is always positive.

Illness is a major alarm for change. It happens to you because it is
needed. It is not the enemy or a monster (I hate how the medical world
sees disease as something to be beaten or conquered). It is an
indication that you have to make different choices. It is a direct
consequence of the choices you have made throughout your life and a
call for change.

That which is greater than us is on your side. It is where this alarm
originates. It (illness) is not an impediment but an opportunity, an
opportunity for growth. In reading this book you are seizing that
opportunity. Opening yourself to a new life, a new phase on your journey.

Be aware that the journey is personal and is only yours. That is why you
have to make choices yourself. Seek guidance, listen to opinions, but

make your own choices. And make them fearlessly. Oftentimes we feel the urge to make a certain choice but then make a different choice out of fear or external pressure. Take time to listen to your inner voice (meditate) and you will always know what choice is right.

I hope you will have understood that life's journey is an all-encompassing experience. It includes your daily actions, what you eat, how you connect with life through wholesome products, how you relate to others, how you love yourself. All of these things are your journey. If you think you are living a good life and you smoke then you aren't. That one event will eventually throw you off in some way.

This doesn't mean that life must be lived in a constant state of strict rules and choices. While you are ill you must be very strict. Once you are healthy it is OK to allow yourself to enjoy a drink, a wonderful dessert or those awesome fries that you enjoy so much; Or to lose sleep because you were out dancing. Just don't harm yourself.

But to engage in addictive behaviors, to abuse in any way, these are the missteps on the journey that will derail you. It is always your choice. No one can stop you except yourself. Any extreme, whether it is physical or spiritual, will affect you adversely.

There is wonder in being alive. Live. Do not take anything for granted. Not a day. Not an act of kindness or the opportunity to give. Make the choice to smile, to reach out, to love, to live in harmony with your environment.

Welcome even illness. See it as a call to change and a chance to grow. Listen to your body as it speaks to you and you will see that this too is a gift, a call to redirect your journey, to find your way to the life you desire. It is an offering to live... to balance your life through necessary change. Or a choice to say goodbye, for this too is a choice you can make.

Death is the inevitable conclusion of life. It should not be forced upon you by illness. But that is your choice. You can die naturally and peacefully or you can die from illness. Illness is not the way to die. Whether you are aware of it or not you have chosen this[35]. You can further choose to continue to its conclusion or you can change.

The change must happen from the core of your being. It is one thing to want to live and a different thing to be afraid to die. They can both look

---

[35] Being born with a life threatening disease is different and a call to a different journey all together.

the same on the outside but on the inside you know the difference. And each one leads to a different journey, each completely acceptable.

So choose your journey. Define a path that is yours and only yours. Take time to 'know' yourself. Then follow your dreams. Choose a life of balance and harmony with nature. Always look inward for direction and to nature for bounty. Live, Laugh, Love...

Appendix A – Preparations

Recipes

I am by no means a cook. While some of these recipes are my own creation many of them have been obtained from sources long forgotten. More importantly my goal is to provide a general guide that will allow you to prepare your own food using ingredients and methods conducive to health. Feel free to research and experiment. The one exception is during the healing process. The nature of illness such as cancer is such that during healing your choices are limited only to those that will facilitate healing.

Guidelines

There are some basic food items that should be a part of a healthy diet and can be added in a variety of ways. Here are the basic preparation instructions for these and ideas on how to use them.

Seaweeds

You should consume seaweed daily during healing and as often as possible as part of your diet. There are many types of seaweeds, mostly sold dry.

Basic Preparation

- Place in a (stainless or ceramic) pan (or a wide pot), cover with water and simmer for about 30 minutes. Add water during simmering, if necessary, as they tend to absorb a lot of water.
- Drain and save the water. I use to make green tea.
- You can then use it in various ways:
  - Season with garlic, ginger, olive oil and other herbs to make a delicious seaweed salad
  - Mix into other recipes such as beans, lentils or rice.

Beans

Beans are a very nutritious food and should be consumed daily. Beans can be purchased canned or dry. Purchase dry beans.

Basic Preparation

- Dry beans must be soaked over night. Place about 1-2 cups in water (in a stainless or ceramic pot) and allow them to sit over night.

- The next day drain the water and refill with fresh water to where the water covers the beans and is about ¼ inch over the top.
- Season the beans. Here is my approach to preparation:
    - 2 tbsp. of cilantro seasoning (recaito)
    - Lots of garlic. I use around 4 tbsp.
    - I like to use cumin as well. To taste.
    - Herbs to taste. You can use a premade mix such as Ms. Dash as long as it doesn't have any additives.
    - You may add sea salt if you like.
- Bring to a boil in a (stainless or ceramic) pot with a lid over medium heat then simmer for about 20 minutes. The beans are done when they 'soften' and the liquid becomes saucy.
- Use in:
    - Mixed with seaweed
    - Mixed with sardines
    - Throw in a few eggs while the beans are simmering for a delicious breakfast treat
    - Mix with rice
    - Mix with vegetables
    - Mash into refried beans (add a little bit of olive oil and lime juice as you mash)
    - Or eat them by themselves

Sprouted Preparation
Sprouted beans are more digestible and nourishing. To sprout:

- Spread dry beans on a large cookie pan. Make sure it is a single layer of beans. They can be close together but not on top of each other.
- Fill with water until the beans are covered.
- Let sit undisturbed until the beans sprout. This is usually about 3 days. When the sprout is about ¼ inch the beans are ready.
- Cook as with basic preparation.

Lentils
Lentils are another great food. The great thing about these is that they are easy to prepare and do not require any softening time as dry beans do.

Basic Preparation
- Place 1-2 cups of dry lentils into a (stainless or ceramic) pot.
- Season them similarly as you would season beans (see above)

- Cover with water, bring to a boil then simmer for about 20 minutes, or until soft.
- Mix with other items just as you would mix beans.

Vegetable/Green Juice

You will find many green juice recipes on the Internet. While this is a great source, many of these juices combine vegetables with fruit (to add flavor), which I consider a no-no. Below is a list of the ingredients that I tend to mix together into the vegetable juices I prepare. This is the result of experimenting over many years. These combinations are easy to prepare and offer great benefits. Use only organic ingredients.

Preparation

I use, and recommend the Vitamixer as the blender to use. I have owned the same unit since 1996 and it still works like new. It is a great investment.

- Basic vegetable mix:
  - Broccoli
  - Mixed greens or Spinach
  - Red cabbage
  - Carrots (small amount)
  - Shiitake mushrooms
  - Cinnamon (1/4 teaspoon)
- Secondary vegetables (as available/on occasion)
  - Spirulina powder (do not use of you are ill)
  - Celery
  - Green beans
  - Avocado
  - Ginger
  - Cucumber
  - Kale
  - Zucchini
  - Bok Choy
- Non vegetable ingredients that I use (required):
  - Flax seed oil with lignans (1 tablespoon)
  - Sulfur crystals (MSM)
- For flavor (if needed):
  - Vanilla extract with Stevia (as much as needed)
  - Pure Cocoa powder
  - Agave (as much as needed)

Place all ingredients in a blender with about 12 oz. of water and a little bit of ice. Blend for about 45-60 seconds, until mixed. IF the drink is too thick either add more water or reduce the amount of vegetables.

These are to be used as indicated in the text.

Lemon/ACV juice
You should take this regularly, upon awakening.

Ingredients
- 1 lemon
- 1 tablespoon organic apple cider vinegar
- 1 cup of water

Preparation
Just mix all the ingredients in a glass and stir.

Anti-parasite tincture
This tincture, now called an anti-parasite tincture, is much more than that. Due to legalities, it cannot be referred to as an anti-illness treatment but that is, in effect, what it is[36].

Ingredients
- Black walnut hull tincture – extra strength
- Clove capsules
- Wormwood capsules

Preparation
The tincture is taken over a 21 day period in quantities as indicated in the following table. It should be taken on an empty stomach upon awakening or right before bed. If you are ill this treatment is required. Note that if you visit the Internet you can read more and learn about alternate ways of using it. This plan here is how I used it[37] and how I've been suggesting it to those I've helped for many years.

Day	Tincture	Wormwood (capsules)	Cloves (capsules)
1	3 drops	2	2
2	4 drops	3	3
3	5 drops	4	4
4	6 drops	5	5

---

[36] This tincture saved my life. When I was sick, taking it marked the turning point towards health.
[37] When I used the tincture resources were limited and I had to figure out what I felt worked. The dosing program outlined has worked very well.

5	7 drops	5	5
6	10 drops	6	6
7	1 teaspoon	6	6
8	1 teaspoon	7	7
9	1 teaspoon	7	7
10	1 teaspoon	7	7
11	1 teaspoon	7	7
12	1 teaspoon	7	7
13		7	7
14	2 teaspoons	7	7
Weekly for a year	2 teaspoons	7	7
Afterwards (indefinitely) Once per month			
1	2 teaspoons	5	5
2	2 teaspoons	6	6
3	2 teaspoons	7	7

Healing Oils

There are 3 oils essential to the healing diet, Flax, Olive and Castor oils. Of these flax and olive oils (extra virgin) should be used in recipes in place of other, potentially damaging, oils. Castor oil, while it can be consumed orally, is used topically.

- Use flax and olive oils, alone or combined, in soups, sauces and salad dressings.
- Take a tablespoon orally, particularly after using a castor oil pack.
- Use olive oil as your cooking oil.

Cereals

The consumption of grains in the diet should be limited. However some grains are OK and are healthy. Here are some of my favorite recipes.

Power Oatmeal

Oatmeal can be particularly helpful to anyone with bowel problems. It can also be very yummy. While consumed mostly at breakfast it can make a great meal any time of day.

Ingredients
- ½ cup of Old fashioned oat meal
- ¼ teaspoon of cinnamon
- ¼ cup raw almonds and walnuts, chopped
- 1 tablespoon of organic, cold pressed, coconut oil
- Agave nectar to taste

- 2 organic eggs
- 1-2 tablespoons of flaxseed oil to taste
- 1-2 scoops vegetarian protein powder (optional)[38]

Preparation

Bring ¾ cups (more or less to taste) of water to a boil. Mix in the oatmeal then simmer for 5 minutes. At the completion of the 5 minutes, mix in the two eggs and simmer for another 1 minute while continuing to mix. Remove from heat and mix in the remaining ingredients.

Seedmeal Delight

Seeds provide an amazing nutritional value. This is one of my favorite seed based cereals. This is very healthy for anyone with bowel/colon problems and should be consumed regularly for those conditions.

Ingredients

- 4 tablespoons of flaxseed
- 4 tablespoons of sunflower seeds
- 4 tablespoons of sesame seeds
- 4 tablespoons of chia seeds
- ¼ teaspoon of cinnamon
- 2-4 tablespoons aloe vera juice to create desired consistency
- 1 tablespoon of flaxseed oil
- Agave nectar to taste
- 100% cocoa powder for chocolate flavoring (if desired)

Preparation

Mix the seeds together and grind in a coffee grinder. Soak over night in the aloe vera juice (refrigerated). Note that the chia seeds are very absorbent. If it looks too dry add more aloe vera juice. When ready to consume mix in the remaining ingredients.

Grains

Grains are a common food source all over the world. However, grains have only been part of the human diet since the advent of agriculture (around 10 thousand years ago). For the most part grains tend to stimulate the body towards bloating and have a tendency to stimulate insulin production.

Having said that the proper consumption of grains, in limited quantities, provides energy and satisfaction. Only grains prepared in accordance

---

[38] I use Naked Pea and Naked Rice protein powders available on amazon.com. This can be used to provide additional protein to the meal.

with the Macrobiotic diet are recommended. There are numerous recipes on the Internet and in the books referenced. One of my favorite is 'The Self-Healing Cookbook' by Kristina Turner.

Seafood
I limit my consumption of animal proteins to no more than once a day[39]. I consume mostly ocean fish baked simply as outlined here. My general rule of thumb is that the fish should be wild caught. There is no telling what types of chemicals are used on farm-raised fish. I do not consume nor do I recommend consuming any kind of fresh water fish as they are all either farmed or from contaminated water.

Baked sea fish (of your choice)
This recipe calls for filleted fish. Generally, you can have it filleted when purchased.

Ingredients
- 1 or more fresh fillets of your chosen fish
- 1-2 tablespoons of olive oil
- Natural herbal seasoning of choice
- Minced garlic to taste (I use about 1 tablespoon per fillet)
- 1 tablespoon of fresh chopped ginger
- 1 tablespoon tamari sauce

Preparation
Coat a flat (stainless or ceramic) pan with olive oil. Place fillets on the pan, then flip, and apply herb seasoning on each side. Sprinkle the tamari sauce over each fillet then sprinkle the minced garlic and ginger on them to taste. Don't over do the ginger!!!!

Preheat oven to 350 degrees. Place the pan with the prepared fillets into the oven and cook for 10-14 minutes depending on the thickness of the fillet. Thin fillets (around ¼ inch) will be ready in about 10 minutes. Thicker fillets under ½ inch should cook for 12 minutes and over ½ inch should cook for about 14 minutes. Check that the inside of the fish is flaky for readiness. Overcooking will dry the fillets.

Serve over a fresh salad or a bed of whole grain rice or with beans (my personal favorite).

---

[39] Humans are not vegetarian. However the modern diet abuses the consumption of animal proteins to the detriment of health and environment. Limit consumption of animal protein.

Sardines

Sardines deserve a special mention. They are one of the most nourishing foods you can consume. You should consume sardines 2-3 times per week.

Most people can only obtain canned sardines. This is one of my exceptions to the 'no canned food' rule. Purchase quality canned sardines if you have no other options. One reason canned is good here is that fresh sardines must be consumed immediately. They don't freeze well and spoil quickly. When purchasing canned sardines (or anything purchased in a can) purchase from different brands as they tend to come from different areas and have a slightly different makeup. There are over 20 varieties of sardines and the areas they come from affect their composition.

Fresh raw sardines are harder to come by. But they are an awesome treat and possibly my favorite food in the whole world (keep reading when you are done laughing…). Purchase only sardines that look fresh and smell good. Avoid bruised or bloated fish. If you have any doubts stick to canned sardines.

Preparation

Scale fresh sardines by rubbing them with your hand over running water. Gut them by holding them belly-up, slicing the belly and using your thumb nail to get rid of the guts. You can eat them with bones as the bones are very small and actually are a source of calcium.

Once ready bake them as you would a thin fish fillet. Keep the seasoning to a minimum. I usually use a little bit of sea salt and lemon juice.

Other sea food

Other types of seafood should be avoided unless you are perfectly healthy. Mussels, clams, oysters, shrimp, squid, octopus are all scavengers. They have great nutritional qualities but may also have varying levels of toxins that are not good for the ill. If you are well feel free to enjoy these items on occasion. Otherwise stay away from them.

Pork

When you are healthy a little bit of pork on occasion can be consumed. I won't elaborate, as there are many cooking methods. Just keep it simple and be sure to use ONLY organic, hormone free pork.

The same holds true for chicken. When you are healthy a little bit of chicken a few times a week is OK. Be sure to use ONLY organic, hormone free chicken. Bake or broil it, grilling and frying should be avoided.

Supplements

As stated in the text, nutritional supplements are essential in today's nutrient depleted world. Here is a list of specific supplements and how to obtain them. Note that not all supplements are created equal. Many have additives that may cause adverse effects. The products recommended all work well as of this writing.

Base/Healing

Supplement	Brand
Co-Enzyme B Complex	Country Life
ALA-ALC (Alpha-lipoic acid, acetyl-l-carnitine)	Vitacost
CoQ10 (100mg)	Dr's Best
Vitamin D3 (5,000 IU)	NOW, Dr's Best
Calcium-Magnesium	NOW
Selenomethionine (200mcg)	Nature's Way, Life Extension
Zinc picolinate (50mg)	NOW
Ester C (500mg)	American Health
Pure Vitamin C powder	Bulk Supplements

Wellness

Supplement	Brand
DHEA (25mg)	LifeExtension
Melatonin 5mg.	NOW
Glucosamine-Chondroitin	Doctor's Best
Chromium polynicotinate (400mcg)	Solgar, Nature's Way

Male

Supplement	Brand
Pygeum-saw palmetto	NOW
L-citruline	Bulk Supplements
L-arginine	Bulk Supplements

Note that as a male I have not had experience to make recommendations for females. I have seen some recommendations, like supplementing iron, not work well. Calcium and Magnesium are both required but are a part of my standard wellness suggestions.

Personal

Personal care should be simple. By using a few basic ingredients you can make a variety of items for personal hygiene that are healthy and produce better results than most commercial products.

Shampoo/soap/ shaving cream

This is simple. Castile soap. It is liquid, long lasting, nourishing and can be used in a variety of ways. As an alternative you can purchase 100% pure soap from a local soap maker. There are sources of pure soap on the Internet as well. If you are ill use only the castile soap until you are well.

Hair conditioner/After-shave

Using hair conditioner and after-shave is not necessary. However, many of us choose to condition our hair and many men use after-shave lotions daily. The best, and most beneficial, conditioner/after-shave that I have ever used (and use to this day) is apple cider vinegar. It's properties and what it does for your hair and skin are nothing short of amazing.

Unlike what many think, the apple cider vinegar is odorless after it dries. It doesn't leave any residue (unlike most commercial hair conditioners) and nourishes both hair and scalp.

It does wonders for the skin, making it an excellent after-shave. I have even used it to remove moles and skin spots.

To use as a hair conditioner or after-shave, mix (organic only) in a container 50/50 with water. Apply it to your hair after shampooing (with castile soap) and leave in for a minute or two, then rinse. As an after-shave apply it to your skin after shaving (it'll sting) and let it dry on the skin. If you have skin spots dab it on them as well and let dry.

Heated castor oil packs use a heating pad to warm a castor oil soaked, wool cloth, allowing the oil to permeate the skin rapidly. It was a common remedy offered in Edgar Cayce's readings[40] for a variety of ailments.

Ingredients
- Electric heating pad (medium size)
- Castor oil (bottle, used over time)
- Uncolored wool[41] cloth (about 20 x 24 inches)
- 1 tablespoon extra virgin olive oil
- 1 large resealable plastic bag (to place the heating pad in)
- 1 large, shallow, rectangular plastic container with lid (to store soaked wool after use)

Preparation
Fold the wool in half two ways, place in the plastic container and soak with castor oil until it is thoroughly saturated. Place the heating pad inside the resealable plastic bag with the electrical cord hanging out.

Lay down comfortable and place the saturated wool directly over the area to be treated. Place the heating pad directly on top of the wool and set it on low heat. After about 5 minutes set it to medium heat or as hot as you can tolerate without getting burned or feeling uncomfortable. Stay this way for the duration of the treatment (around 20-30 minutes).

When time is up, store the wool in the plastic container. Clean the area with a wet, warm towel. Consume the tablespoon of olive oil.

Toothpaste

I brush my teeth simply by dabbing a little bit of baking soda (about ¼ teaspoon) on my toothbrush, brushing for about a minute, then rinsing. I follow that with 5 drops of 35% food grade peroxide on my toothbrush (which debacterializes it), brushing for another 30 seconds. DO NOT rinse after brushing with the peroxide.

If you prefer more traditional toothpaste try the following recipe. You should still brush with the 35% food grade peroxide at least once a day.

---

[40] Refer to the reference section for resources that speak about Edgar Cayce and his famous readings.
[41] If you are allergic to wool it is OK to substitute cotton. The wool lasts much longer and allows the oil to flow better.

Homemade Peppermint and Coconut Oil Toothpaste

Ingredients
- 1/2 cup bentonite clay
- 2 tsp. baking soda
- 2/3 cup water
- 1/4 cup coconut oil
- 8 drops peppermint essential oil

Preparation
Mix the ingredients in a bowl. Mix until it forms a paste. Store it in a jar with a lid. To use it spoon some onto your toothbrush using a small spoon. Dampen the paste by putting your brush under some gently running water. Brush as usual.

Other useful remedies
There are a few other remedies that I have used very successfully that may be helpful to you.

Colon cleanse
If you are ill, use this remedy regularly. If you have any type of colon related disease use this daily.

Ingredients
- ½ cup aloe vera gel
- ½ cup purified water
- 1 tablespoon chia seeds
- 1 tablespoon cold pressed, virgin coconut oil
- 1 tablespoon flaxseed oil with lignans

Preparation
Mix all ingredients together in a blender. Drink slowly, preferably on an empty stomach.

Essential oils
Essential oils have a variety of uses and healing properties. Here are some excellent remedies that you can use in a variety of circumstances. Note that the quality of the oil is extremely important. Purchase oils from a reputable source.

For more details go online and search under 'aromatherapy' or 'essential oil uses'. I've used the following and can attest to their efficacy.

Treating skin spots/acne/sores/boils/psoriasis/toe fungus/ringworm
Use before bed by applying it directly to the affected area. If you feel it is too strong you can mix it with witch hazel.

Dandruff/lice
Use on your scalp by mixing as follows:

Ingredients
- 2 tablespoons aloe vera gel
- 10 drops lavender essential oil
- 25 drops tea tree essential oil
- 1 teaspoon coconut oil

Preparation
Mix all ingredients together and rub into your scalp. Let it sit for about 10 minutes (or longer) then shampoo off.

Household
The following remedies are easy to make and will meet practically every need you have around the home. For further information and other remedies check the references in Appendix C.

Kitchen Surface Cleansers
Kitchen surfaces are major centers for bacteria formation and contaminants, particularly if they are cleaned with commercial products. Here are a few of my personal remedies.

For stainless surfaces, glass stove tops, or oven surfaces:

Surface scrub Preparation
Mix a little bit of olive oil with baking soda to form a paste.

Use a mild scrubbing pad. Finish with a liquid mix of distilled white vinegar and lemon juice in water. Wipe dry.

For counter tops just use the liquid mix of vinegar, lemon juice and water.

Ingredients
- 2 cups of water
- Juice of one large lemon or two small ones
- ¼ cup of distilled white vinegar

Preparation

Mix all ingredients together and place in a spray bottle.

Bathroom Scum Removal

A strong mix of white distilled vinegar and water (50/50) in a spray bottle sprayed on the surface scum and allowed to sit for a few minutes will soften water residue. Add baking soda to make a scrubbing compound as needed. To do this just spray the area first and after a minute or two place some baking soda directly on a scrubbing pad and rub down.

Air freshener

Keeping your home smelling fresh can be done in a variety of ways. Try a few of these until you find what works for you.

Essential Oil Diffuser

Simple oil diffusers are available in most places that sell candles. My favorites use a little bit of candle wax (about 2 tablespoons) melted over a candle with a few drops (10-15) of your favorite essential oil(s) mixed in. Refresh with more essential oil as needed.

Spray Freshener

There are many recipes for healthy spray fresheners. Here is one of my favorites. You can go online and look for other recipes and ideas.

Ingredients
- 1 ½ cups of water
- 5 sticks dried cinnamon sticks
- 2 tablespoons of dried basil
- 10 drops of lavender or lemon essential oil (try them both)
- 1 tablespoon witch hazel

Preparation

Bring water to a boil then mix all ingredients together in a stainless pot. Turn off the heat and allow the mixture to steep and cool down. Mix it a few times while the water is still hot. Once cool, filter through a fine mesh (or a coffee filter) and pour into a spray bottle. Shake before each use.

Laundry Detergent

Your clothing is in contact with your skin all day and your bed sheets all night. Your skin absorbs what is on it. It is important to have toxin free clothing (be aware of wrinkle free, never iron and man made fabrics). Your laundry detergent can be a major source of toxicity. Here is my laundry detergent recipe.

Ingredients
- 2 cups of borax powder
- 2 cups of washing soda
- ¼ cup baking soda
- Dr. Bronner's bar soap

Preparation
Pulverize the bar soap using a fine grater or a food processor. Mix with the remaining ingredients and store in a cool dry location. Use about ¼ to ½ cup per load, depending on load size.

Wood/Tile Floor Cleaner
Clean, toxin free floors are important for health. I walk around the house barefoot (walking barefoot is very good for you). If you have small children it is even more important to be chemical/toxin free.

Ingredients
- 2 cups of distilled white vinegar
- 1 gallon of hot water
- 2 tablespoons of liquid castile soap
- 2 tablespoons of olive oil

Preparation
Mix all ingredients into a mop bucket. Mop the floor as usual.

Appendix B – Physical Exercises

Exercise Descriptions

The following paragraphs describe the exercises mentioned in the text. It is possible to find descriptions and videos on the Internet. If you do this be careful as many online descriptions may be slightly different than those described here. In particular, pay attention to:

- **Breathing patterns**
  In general you exhale when you exert force (contract) and inhale when you extend. There are exceptions so please be aware of the pattern. I have seen many instructions online that state incorrect breathing patterns or don't state them at all.

- **Execution speed**
  Most exercises online are executed much faster than I would suggest. All movements should be slow and deliberate. If you notice I specify how long it should take to perform each repetition. This is VERY important.

Cyclist's bends
This exercise works the entire spinal column. It should be performed very slowly and deliberately with care and attention to form. There should be no pain whatsoever.

1. Sit on the floor by getting on your knees. Keep your legs together and rest your buttock on the heels of you feet.

2. Clasp your hands behind your head and keep your elbows out.

3. As you exhale, curl your spine down towards the floor starting from your neck and working downward. It should take you about 5-6 seconds to exhale completely and reach the bottom.

4. Without resting your head, reverse the action as you inhale, slowly straightening your spine from the bottom up towards your neck as you come up. Again, move slowly, taking about 5-6 seconds to come up.

5. Repeat the movement, synchronized with your breathing. Aim for 12 repetitions. As you get stronger, go slower, taking about 10 seconds in each direction.

Abdominal crunches
Do this movement using a 'bosu' ball (or you can use an exercise ball if you have one).

1. Lay with your lower back on the ball. Your hips should be over the side.

2. As you exhale, crunch your abdomen by moving your torso up, pointing your arms/hands straight over your head, and curling your hips upwards as in a slow pelvic thrust. Do this slowly, taking about 4 seconds to complete the crunch.

3. As you inhale bring yourself back, stretching slightly over the ball while keeping your arms overhead.

4. Repeat the movement, synchronized with your breathing. Aim for 20-50 repetitions depending on your strength level. Do not over exert yourself.

Side twists
Do this movement using a 'bosu' ball (or you can use an exercise ball if you have one).

1. Lay with your lower back on the ball. Your hips should be over the side.

2. Clasp your hands behind your head. As you exhale, curl forward in a small arc, bringing your right elbow over to your left side towards your left knee (without straining). Do this slowly, taking about 2 seconds to complete the movement.

3. As you inhale bring yourself back to the starting position.

4. Without pausing, repeat the movement, this time bringing your left elbow over to your right side towards your right knee.

5. Aim to do 20-50 repetitions (10-25 to each side).

Simple squat
Do this movement taking care not to hurt yourself. If you are not accustomed to exercising, your legs are likely to be weak. Build yourself up slowly. If you need support you can place your hands on your knees or hold on to the back of a chair.

1. Start by standing with your legs shoulder width apart.

2. As you inhale, squat slowly while keeping your back straight and looking straight forward.

3. You should squat until your thighs are parallel to the floor. If it first this is difficult squat as low as you can without feeling any discomfort.

4. Squat slowly, taking from 2-5 seconds to lower yourself to where your thighs are parallel to the floor. As you get stronger aim for 10 seconds.

5. As you exhale, bring yourself back to a standing position. Do so slowly, taking 2-5 seconds to come back to a standing position.

6. Repeat in a continuous motion (without resting at the top) aiming for 20 repetitions.

Single leg heel raise

If you are weak you may do this exercises with both legs until you get stronger. Use a wood block (or a yoga block) with a rounded edge or stair step to raise your toes on.

1. Place the ball of your foot on the wood block and stretch your heel towards the floor.

2. Slowly raise your heel until you are on your toe tips (on the wood block).

3. Without pausing, bring your heel back down slowly.

4. Repeat in a continuous motion. Aim for 20 repetitions (for each leg). As you get stronger do the movement slower, until it takes you about 10 seconds each way.

Kettle bell swing

This is one of the best overall movements you can perform. At first, do it slowly so as to not hurt yourself. It will strengthen you quickly. The downside is that you will need a kettle bell (or a dumbbell).

If you are weak (or recovering from a back injury), start without the kettle bell. As you build strength build up the weight. A fit male should be using around 50lbs. A fit female should be using around 40lbs.

1. Start with a wide leg stance with the kettle bell on the floor between your legs.

2. While keeping your back straight and knees slightly bent, reach down and grab the kettle bell.

3. As you inhale, using your torso bring the kettle bell up in front of you in a swinging motion.

4. At the top of the swing contract your buttocks with your back straight.

5. While exhaling, bring the kettle bell down without touching the floor.

6. Repeat as a continuous motion, synchronized with your breath. Aim for 50 repetitions. At first you may only be able to do a few so work your way up slowly, making sure not to hurt yourself.

Wide hand pushup
This classic is an excellent movement for building upper body strength. You will likely have to start very slowly. At first you may have to do them with your weight on your hands and knees. When you are stronger you can progress to hands and toes. Use a set of wood blocks (or yoga blocks) for your hands.

1. Start by placing your hands on wood blocks slightly further than shoulder width apart and your legs straight out behind you with your weight on the balls of your feet (or knees) such that your body is straight from head to heel (this is called a plank position).

2. While inhaling, slowly lower your torso towards the floor, taking care to keep your body straight and aligned, like a plank.

3. Before reaching the floor, exhale and bring your torso back up until your arms are straight but without locking your elbows.

4. Repeat as a continuous motion, synchronized with your breath. Aim for 12 repetitions, taking about 10 seconds while going down. Ideally you would do 10 seconds going up as well but this is very difficult. Do your best.

Wide grip pull-up (palms facing away)
This classic movement complements the push up and makes for one of the best upper body strength building exercises ever. To do this you will need a bar to pull up from. If you do not have a bar you can obtain one by installing a doorway pull-up bar. You will also likely need a stool to

support yourself as you will more than likely not be able to pull up your full body weight (most people can't. This is OK).

If you are ill you may not be able to do this exercise. If this is the case the use of a physical rehabilitation facility or a gym can help you. And you should seek the help, as it is important to your wellbeing.

1. Start by grabbing the bar with palms facing out and slightly wider than shoulder width apart.

2. Place your feet on a stool to support your weight.

3. As you exhale, pull yourself up until your chin is over the pull-up bar. Use your legs to help you up (by pushing) if needed, but as little as possible.

4. As you inhale, lower yourself slowly, taking between 2-6 seconds to lower your body. Do not lock your elbows.

5. Repeat the movement, synchronized with your breath. Aim for 8 repetitions.

Lateral raise (with weights or exercise bands)
This movement strengthens the shoulders. If you have weights you can use those. A pair of 5 or 10lb dumbbells are usually enough (If you are fit you can use heavier weights). Or you can use exercise bands as well.

1. Start by standing and holding a dumbbell in each hand, or, if you are using an exercise band by holding the band with an end in each hand and pinning the center under your feet.

2. As you exhale, and with elbows slightly bent, raise your arms laterally until they are slightly above your shoulders.

3. While inhaling, slowly (3-10 seconds) lower your arms until they are a few inches from your sides.

4. Repeat as a continuous motion, synchronized with your breathing. Aim for 8-12 repetitions, lowering as slow as possible on each repetition.

Iso-tension arm curl/extension
This exercise is performed without any weight, totally dependent on your

arm antagonistic muscles (bicep/triceps) and mental focus. It is a simple movement that requires a strong focus to perform properly.

1. Start with your arms at your sides.

2. As you exhale, create tension in your upper arms by tensioning both bicep and triceps.

3. While holding this tension curl your arm, resisting the curling motion antagonistically and taking about 5 seconds to complete the curl. Focus on your bicep (the muscle on the front of your arm).

4. Without releasing the tension, extend your arms (keep them at your sides) slowly (taking about 5 seconds), focusing on contracting your triceps.

5. Repeat as a continuous motion, synchronized with your breathing. Repeat 8-10 times, keeping a strong focus throughout the entire movement.

Appendix C – References

Books

Following is a list of books that have influenced and contributed to my journey and the book you are holding. They're in no particular order and are listed here for those of you that like to read and are curious to know more.

Title	Author
The Untethered Soul	Michael Singer
Never Be Sick Again	Raymond Francis
The Biology of Belief	Dr. Bruce Lipton
The Self-Healing Cookbook	Kristina Turner
The Power of Touch	Phyllis R. Davis, PhD
Touching	Ashley Montagu
The Cure for All Cancers	Dr. Hulda Clarke
The Oil-Protein Diet	Dr. Johanna Budwig
The Cancer Prevention Diet	Michio Kushi
Quantum Healing	Deepak Chopra
Secrets of Your Cells	Sondra Barrett, PhD
Detecting Your Hidden Allergies	Dr. William G. Crook, M.D.
The Hidden Messages in Water	Masaru Emoto
The New Nutrition	Dr. Michael Colgan
The 4 Hour Body	Tim Ferris
Your Body Believes Every Word You Say	Barbara Hoberman Levine
Home Safe Home	Debra Lynn Dadd
How to Grow Fresh Air	Dr. B. C. Wolverton
You Already Know What To Do	Sharon Franquemont
Ayurveda	Dr. Vasant Lad
Instant Self Hypnosis	Forbes Robbins Blair
Conscious Breathing	Gay Hendricks, PhD
The Heart Speaks	Mimi Guarneri, M.D.
Secrets of Longevity	Dr. Maoshing Ni
Somatic Patterning	Mary Ann Foster
Self-Healing	Meir Schneider
Healing Mind, Body & Spirit	M. J. Abadie

Websites

These are some websites that have content that may be helpful to those reading this book. I do not necessarily agree or endorse everything stated here so please use your own judgment in making use of what is stated.

SITE URL	CONTENT
www.amazon.com	Purchase supplements/books
www.bodyecology.com	
www.fourhourbody.com	
www.4hourlife.com	
www.vitamix.com	Purchase the Vitamix blender (recommended: C-5200)
www.dharmacrafts.com	Yoga/meditation gear
www.drclark.com	Learn about Hulda Clark's great work.
www.drclarkestore.com	Purchase tincture and other nutrients
www.macrobiotics.org.uk/recipes	Recipes for eating well
http://liveenergized.com/category/alkaline-recipes/	More recipes for healthy eating
www.home-safe-home.org/	Safety against home toxicity/chemicals
www.wellnessmama.com	Health remedies
www.innerengineering.com	Self growth, relationships
https://www.psychologytoday.com/blog/rewire-your-brain-love/200911/nine-ways-meditating-brain-creates-better-relationships	Meditation and relationships
https://www.mountainroseherbs.com/catalog/aromatherapy/essential-oils	Essential oil purchase
http://www.planttherapy.com/	Essential oil purchase
http://www.edgarcayce.org/	The Edgar Cayce website

Resources

The following resources, primarily interviews and documentaries, are also of great value in understanding the path to health and healing. Most of these can be found on Netflix or on Amazon Videos.

URL	Content
www.youtube.com/watch?v=jjj0xVM4x1I	Video of Bruce Lipton discussing Biology of Belief. He has other great links as well.
www.youtube.com/watch?v=2_6ad9URawc	Michael Singer on Mindfulness.
www.youtube.com/watch?v=EJt4iMmqhpY	Raymond Francis video, Never be Sick Again
Food, Inc.	Documentary on the fiasco of the food industry.
Cut Poison Burn	The facts around medical cancer treatment (and why it is killing you)

Fed Up	Documentary about how the system contributes to our dietary issues
Cowspiracy	The truth about sustainability and global warming.
Crazy Sexy Cancer	An inspiring story about how cancer changes lives and how it can teach us to live.
The Gerson Miracle	Gerson therapy and why it works.
Forks Over Knives	How our modern foods contributes to disease.
Food Matters	"
Fresh, The Movie	Fresh food and what is being done about it.
The Future of Food	The scary direction that the food industry is taking if we don't change it.
Fat, Sick and Nearly Dead	An inspiring story of dietary change and survival.
Numen, The Nature of Plants	Why plants matter to health and how conventional healthcare is killing us
Dirt! The Movie	The importance of soil in life.
Doctored	The deceit of doctors and modern medicine.
Bag It, the movie	The danger and destructive nature of plastics
Tapped	The bottled water industry and it's destruction of life.
Bought	The conspiracy of food, drugs, health insurance and vaccines.

Appendix D – Addiction/Recovery

I have added this Appendix due to the increasing rates of addiction that begin through medical channels. My experience with addiction is limited as this is not my focus. I have learned a few things over time and feel that it is important to address the issue. If you are suffering from an addiction, use this only as a starting point.

It is unfortunate that the pain caused by illness often causes addiction to painkillers. When we are in pain our biggest desire is for the pain to go away. Often, the pain is emotional. It is a pain associated with missing connectedness to others and the world. This leads to prescription painkillers, some very effective... and addictive.

As a result there are many cases where illness leads to addiction. It starts off with painkillers such as oxy or hydrocodone (opiates) and eventually turns into heroin when it is no longer possible to get prescriptions[42]. In an effort to get away from the dangers of heroin (and street drugs) the user turns to methadone, legal and possibly the most dangerous of all the opiates.

These aren't the only addictive drugs. Xanax and other depressants as well as stimulants (amphetamines), while not as deadly are also common. It is sad to see how drugs, possibly intended to help, end up becoming detrimental and even fatal to their users.

This Appendix is a summary of what I have learned by helping others off of these dangerous killers. If you or someone you know is suffering from an addiction read on.

My experience has been mostly with opiates, which cause pain relief by producing dopamine (the human 'feel good' hormone). These drugs become addictive very quickly, as the body stops producing its own dopamine when they are used for more than a few days.

Eventually, the user attempts to get off the drug. And this itself is very painful, leading to the use of more drugs, in an endless cycle of pain avoidance.

---

[42] In the US more people die from prescription opiate overdoses than from heroin and cocaine combined.

There is a large pool of evidence that shows addictive

> "The opposite of addiction is not sobriety, it is human connection."
> Johann Hari

behavior is caused by psychological emptiness, the lack of connection to others and purpose in life. In the end humans are bonding creatures, and when we are not bonding, as we should, when our lives lack direction and human support, we suffer... and often wind up seeking the short-term satisfaction offered by addiction.

So my experience is that addiction cannot be ended medically, by just removing the drug. This may work in the short term but eventually there is a relapse, a return to the short-term fulfillment that at least temporarily alleviates the empty void left by the missing human connections and purpose in life. Addiction is a disease, a disease of the human spirit, of a human being who's been denied the basic tenets of being human, and has broken down as a result.

The breaking point that leads to addiction is different for each person. Some people need more connection and bonding than others. I've concluded that this is because some of us have a stronger inner resiliency and self-connection. This inner resiliency is usually seen in people that meditate and have learned to quiet the mind. The inner peace bought about by a quiet mind connects us in a different way.

So addressing addiction requires filling the human need to bond and have purpose. As this is addressed the addiction itself is then addressed.

As stated, my exposure to addiction recovery has been limited to the cases that I've worked with. I think the pattern is similar whether you are addicted to drugs, alcohol, cigarettes or gambling.

- Physically, you must take care of yourself. Following the guidelines in this book accomplishes this.
- Mentally, you must focus on yourself.
  - Understand what you want from your life. What do you like to do and what are you good at? What do you dream of?
  - Connect with your loved ones. Parental bonds, siblings, close friends. Reach out and help others.
  - Take time each day to meditate and find your inner rhythm.

o Do not get discouraged. Do not lose hope. Remember that anything in life worth doing requires discipline.

Once you have a plan around the above you are ready to confront your addiction. You will find that when you are truly supported your addictive behaviors will start to go away. They may not disappear immediately, particularly if you've been addicted for a long time.

Usually, the easiest way to address addiction is to down dose over a predetermined period of time. This is true for physical addictions. Mental addictions can be overcome by disconnecting yourself from the source of the addiction.

Support

Support groups can be very helpful. However, they can also be very dangerous. Some support groups advocate thinking processes that are hurtful and not based on a true understanding of addiction, IMO. A good support group is:

- Led by qualified professionals
- Has a track record for helping others
- Makes you feel good and accepted (not little and victimized, your addiction is NOT bigger than you)
- Has counselors that themselves are recovering and understand your challenges

Often your best advisor is someone that has been where you are and is well aware of what you are going through. You should feel a sense of compassion and empathy within the group. Any group that blindly advocates cold turkey, is overly religious, uses negativity (makes you feel unworthy) is not likely going to be helpful.

I have seen some amazing support programs that do more than sit around and talk. Look for empowerment, a group that looks to provide you with resources and direction. The group should focus on you and not on any agenda or self-promotion.

Opiates

Opiates are the most common addictive killers. More and more they have their root in prescription painkillers. Our medical system does very little to reinstate the health of addictions caused by the system. Opiates are also very effective at alleviating the pain caused by human emptiness, becoming a very difficult addiction to overcome.

Here I will address overcoming the physical addiction. These are broken down into two sections, non-methadone and methadone based.

Methadone is possibly the strongest opiate of all. It is legal and used as an alternative to acquiring opiates on the street (heroin, hydros, roxys). But it creates a dependency that is very difficult to overcome. I have heard it referred to as 'liquid handcuffs' and that is true. It is a business, albeit a legal one, and its use is on the rise as many people that get on never get off (yes, methadone users tend to use it for life). Withdrawal from methadone is long and painful. It allows you to function 'normally' so it is often considered a good alternative to other opiates. I disagree with this. If you are considering methadone but have not yet started my advice is DON'T DO IT. It is easier to detox and get off any other opiate.

Non-methadone detox

- Follow the guidelines in this book for a healthy lifestyle.
- Get the support of friends and family and/or a support group.
- Establish a plan for down dosing from your opiates:
  - Dose down to a minimal dose over a 30 day period
  - Bring the dose down as fast as you can tolerate. You will not feel well during this time. The goal is to be able to function. I good indicator is sleep. As long as you are not losing sleep you are down dosing effectively.
- Purchase and consume the following supplements for the next 30 days:
  - Elimitrol (Day and Night)
  - Omega 3-6-9 (morning and evening)
  - (morning, mid-day, afternoon, evening):
    - 5-HTP (morning, mid-day, afternoon, evening)
    - L-tyrosine
    - L-phenadrine
  - Liquid kava-kava (bedtime)
  - Melatonin (bedtime)
- Start your detox on a Friday. If you work you can work that day even though you will start to feel pretty lousy.
- Stick with it. The next few days will be very difficult. Enlist the support of your loved ones to help you.
- If they work for you try using sleeping aids. Try to sleep it off as much as possible (you will feel exhausted but sleep will be difficult)
- Drink at least a glass of water per hour
- By Monday you should feel better. Stay home and try to sleep.

- You should start feeling more functional by Tuesday. You're passed the worse part and your body is now returning to normal.

After this the goal is now to stay away from the opiates. You will be tempted and you will have cravings. This will continue for the next few months but will become better and better every day. This is where support and bonding pull you through. It is the beginning of a better life and a time to focus your attention on what you want to do for yourself.

Methadone Detox

If you are on methadone you must be more patient. It will take more time to rid you of your dependency due to the extended effects of methadone. There are treatment centers that can help you detox faster. Essentially they take you off the opiate, use medication to alleviate symptoms and sedate you for a few days while you get over it. They are expensive but work if you choose to take that route. Otherwise you can detox over a period of a few months as follows:

- Follow the guidelines in this book for a healthy lifestyle.
- Get the support of friends and family and/or a support group.
- Establish a plan for dosing down from your opiates:
  - Dose down to a minimal dose over a 30-90 day period depending on your current dose. Methadone is dosed anywhere from 25mg to 80mg. Start dosing down at the rate of 5mg per week until you are at 25mg. Stay at 25mg for 2 weeks. At this point you may have to consult with the clinic to continue dosing down. They should help you to continue until you are at a minimal dose of about 5mg.
  - You will not feel well during this time. The goal is to be able to function. I good indicator is sleep. As long as you are not losing sleep you are down dosing effectively.
- Purchase and consume the following supplements for the next 30 days:
  - Elimitrol (Day and Night)
  - Omega 3-6-9 (morning and evening)
  - (morning, mid-day, afternoon, evening):
    - 5-HTP (morning, mid-day, afternoon, evening)
    - L-tyrosine
    - L-phenadrine
  - Liquid kava-kava (bedtime)
  - Melatonin (bedtime)

- Start your detox on a Friday. If you work you can work that day even though you will start to feel pretty lousy.
- Stick with it. You will need about a week to get off methadone's effects. These days will be difficult but should be tolerable and you should start to feel better after the 3rd day. Enlist the support of your loved ones to help you. If you work you should take this week off.
- If they work for you try using sleeping aids. Try to sleep it off as much as possible (you will feel exhausted but sleep will be difficult). If you have access to a doctor a prescription sleep aid is useful here.
- Drink at least a glass of water per hour.
- By Monday you should start feeling better. Stay home and try to sleep.
- With methadone you may not start feeling functional until later in the week.
- It will take a few weeks for the methadone effects to be completely gone. You should be able to function after the first week.

Getting off methadone is probably the hardest thing you'll have to do. But it is worth it.

Non-Opiates
Getting off of non-opiates is similar to getting off opiates. You should follow those guidelines noting that:

- Dosing down is the least painful method, especially if you are on high doses.
- If you are addicted to Xanax you should detox slowly, following the guidelines for methadone detox.
  - Depending on how much you are taking and how long you've been taking it, it may be a good idea to detox with the help of a doctor.
  - Pay attention to mental symptoms:
    - Anxiety
    - Panic
    - Hallucination
    - Moodiness
  - If you are using it to avoid life circumstances that cause anxiety or other stresses you should address those first as relapse is very likely when you confront them.

- Sunshine helps. If you live in an area where you can have daily sun exposure do so. Be sure to use adequate sun protection.
- Crystal meth addiction should be done carefully. Be aware that:
  - You may feel depressed and suicidal. For this reason you should have 24x7 support from a friend or partner.
  - Cravings can last for extended periods. Crystal meth damages the brain and dopamine receptors.
  - Follow the methadone detox steps.
  - You will need a strong support network, as cravings can be very intense due to bouts of depression and anxiety.
- Find a focus. Music or even taking up a sport can be very helpful. Learning new skills will also engage the brain and help significantly.

Regardless of your addiction it is important to find the underlying motives that make you do what you do. These must be addressed so that your life itself nurtures you and provides you with all the dopamine (the hormone that most drugs increase) you can ever want.

Books
The following books are amazing when it comes to understanding and overcoming addictive behaviors.

Title	Author
Chasing The Scream	Johann Hari
Recover!	Stanton Peele, Ph. D. & Ilse Thompson